Living with Chronic Disease: Measuring Important Patient-Reported Outcomes

Paul Kamudoni
Nutjaree Johns
Sam Salek

Living with Chronic Disease: Measuring Important Patient-Reported Outcomes

University of Hertfordshire UH
Adis
KHON KAEN UNIVERSITY
IMD Institute of Medicine Development

Paul Kamudoni
Global Evidence & Value Development –
R&D, Merck KgaA
Darmstadt
Germany

Nutjaree Johns
Faculty of Pharmaceutical Sciences
Khon Kaen University
Khon Kaen
Thailand

Institute of Medicines Development
Cardiff
United Kingdom

Sam Salek
School of Life & Medical Sciences
University of Hertfordshire
Hatfield
Hertfordshire
United Kingdom

ISBN 978-981-13-4143-4 ISBN 978-981-10-8414-0 (eBook)
https://doi.org/10.1007/978-981-10-8414-0

Softcover re-print of the Hardcover 1st edition 2018

Printed on acid-free paper

This Adis imprint is published by the registered company Springer Nature Singapore Pte Ltd.
The registered company address is: 152 Beach Road, #21-01/04 Gateway East, Singapore 189721, Singapore

Foreword

We live in an era of exciting discovery and innovation in biomedical science and technology. The resulting medical breakthroughs are providing safe and effective treatments for often serious and life-threatening diseases and are thus transforming lives. Notwithstanding and often because of this progress, the number of patients living with chronic disease continues to grow.

A recent analysis by the Global Burden of Disease Study (GBD) found that although death rates for most causes have declined worldwide since 1990, there has not been a similar decline in age-standardized years lived with disability (YLD) rates. For many causes, YLD rates have either remained the same or have increased, and the increasing prevalence of disabling disease produces increased demand for health system services.[1] Health care for patients with chronic disease now accounts for an increasing share of overall health spending. A recent study by the Rand Corporation[2] found, for example, that 60% of American adults live with at least one chronic condition and account for 90% of US health care spending, and the estimated 28% of Americans who are living with three or more chronic conditions account for as much as 67% of US health spending.

The realities of growing disease prevalence, and finite resources available to responsible jurisdictions to treat patients living with chronic disease, may present a limited horizon of rewards to innovators just as it presents continuing challenges for health care payers. Fortunately, in parallel with these burgeoning challenges there is an increasing recognition that patients living with chronic disease have special expertise and a critical role to play in identifying what is most meaningful and could inform the assessment of value.

As part of a commitment made under its 2012 prescription drug user fee reauthorization, FDA conducted over twenty patient-focused meetings each involving a different disease area and patient community. These meetings, in which patients directly discussed the impact of disease on their daily life, and the burden of current treatments, provided new insights for FDA reviewers and reinforced the importance

[1] Global Burden of Disease Study 2016 Collaborators (Sept. 2017) Global, regional, and national incidence, prevalence, and years lived with disability for 328 diseases and injuries for 195 countries, 1990–2016: a systematic analysis for the Global Burden of Disease Study 2016. Lancet 390(10100):1211–1259

[2] Buttorff C, Ruder T, Bauman M (2017) Multiple chronic conditions in the United States, Rand Corporation. https://www.rand.org/pubs/tools/TL221.html

of early exploration and incorporation of the patient's experience to inform drug development, particularly for chronic conditions. The patient's perspective can not only inform overall framing of the assessment of drug benefit and risk but also provide a more direct source of evidence regarding the benefits and risks. This can be achieved if methodologically sound data collection tools, typically involving patient-reported outcomes (PROs), are developed and deployed within clinical studies of an investigational therapy. If such evidence could be more routinely used as a basis for regulatory assessment of drug benefits and risks, it could be incorporated in drug labeling to better inform decisions by doctors and patients at the point of care. This evidence could also inform estimates of a new treatment impact on the quality of life and other considerations for health technology assessors and payers' decision making.

In addition, early and continued attention and measurement of what matters to patients may offer other benefits for drug developers. Clinical trials that are designed and conducted to account for patients' perspectives on eligibility criteria, trial site accessibility, and tolerability of planned procedures are more likely to achieve desired levels of enrollment and higher retention among participants, thus reducing problems of study delay and missing data. Medicines that are designed to improve tolerability and otherwise reduce treatment burden are also likely to enable better patient adherence and associated clinical benefit.

For some, the promise of all these benefits may be tempered by perceived risks of undertaking development of PROs. The development process outlined in some of the literature and earlier regulatory guidance may seem to suggest striving for an ideal that may be difficult to achieve. Some drug sponsors and researchers have expressed concern about the potentially high cost and uncertain benefits of de novo development of PROs. Continued uncertainty may limit the interest of researchers and industry to engage in this important work. Inconsistent quality in PROs, another potential by-product of uncertainty about standards and approaches, will both limit the utility for decision makers and generally undercut confidence in these data despite their potential to improve development and delivery of treatments for patients. To help address these concerns FDA is currently taking steps including development of new guidance to better integrate the patient's experience in drug development. Success and sustainability will require development of a more standardized practical approach that provides predictability and the rigor needed to generate quality data for decision making.

Recognizing the need this book provides both a conceptual foundation and a well-described approach to the development and use of PROs. The authors provide a step-by-step approach that addresses both important methodological and practical considerations for conducting this work. Further clarity is provided by use of a case study based on the chronic condition of hyperhidrosis. This book provides an important contribution at an opportune time. The role of patient advocacy groups and engagement with patients has never been greater, and interest in the use of PROs is growing, but resources and experience with PRO work among drug developers and others remain limited. The authors provide a clear and practical path forward.

Beltsville, MD, USA Theresa Mullin

Preface

The field of patient-reported outcomes (PRO) measurement is undergoing dramatic transformation, encompassing the development as well as application of PRO measures in different contexts. The rigorous and accurate measurement of PROs in clinical practice or medicines development programmes is now considered a need, from the patient's perspective, and a requirement, from the perspective of health authorities. For example, in the UK, the NHS is rolling out routine assessment of certain PROs for all patients undergoing certain surgical intervention, pre- and post-surgery. Demonstration of benefits in terms of patient-relevant outcomes is required for medicines undergoing benefit-risk assessment as part of health technology assessments in Germany. This raises the important question—where are we in the transition of the field from an art to a hard science?

This book was born out of a belief that the recent developments have catapulted (or fast-tracked the progress of) PRO measurement into a mature science, given the research and application experience accumulated, requiring a streamlined framework and practical guidance. While numerous textbooks have been published on the topic of PRO measurement recently, we wanted to offer one that would be highly practical as a guide, showing the step-by-step considerations and activities, involved in conceptualizing, developing and applying PRO measures, using our own research work as a case study.

We propose an 8-step roadmap for development of a PRO measure:

- Step 1—Define objectives of development of the PRO measure
- Step 2—Generate hypothesis and conceptualise the PRO measure: disease model/hypothetical conceptual physico-psychosocial model
- Step 3—Gather and select item concepts: concept elicitation/qualitative research
- Step 4—Design and build the PRO measure: content definition/item generation
- Step 5—Refine the PRO measure's content: cognitive debriefing/content validation panels
- Step 6—Explore the PRO measure's practicality and applicability
- Step 7—Fine-tune the PRO measure, evaluate item performance, establish scoring algorithms
- Step 8—Generate psychometric evidence and other supportive information

As part of the new roadmap, we identify how innovative approaches should be incorporated in each of the steps, including how patients and other key stakeholders could be engaged in the research process. We have devoted a good portion of the book to illustrating the new roadmap using a PRO measure development programme in dermatology in which we were involved. Such case study allowed us to go into detail: describing decisions made at key steps of the PRO development process; our rationale and practical considerations at each point; and how we, ultimately, executed our research strategy. Thus, we have been able to fully illustrate how the proposed roadmap could actually be realized.

Given the increasingly diverse purposes and settings for assessing PROs, this book has also addressed the topic of how to integrate PRO assessments in routine clinical practice, clinical research and medicines development programmes. Much of the material presented for this section is based on our research integrating PRO assessments in palliative clinics, as well as one-to-one interviews on the concept of PROs with executives working in the pharmaceutical industry and medicine regulatory agencies.

The book is organized under 7 chapters. Chapter 1 lays the foundation, setting the aims and objectives of the book and discussing the rationale, role and importance of assessing PROs in chronic conditions. In Chapter 2, the new PRO roadmap is presented. This is then illustrated in Chapters 3–6 using a case study research in dermatology. This includes how information from literature review was summarized into a conceptual model and qualitative research carried out to capture patients' experience of the disease under investigation, in Chapter 3; drafting of new PRO measures and confirmation of content validity engaging patients and clinicians, in Chapter 4; use of modern test methods (i.e. item response theory) to fine-tune PRO measures, in Chapter 5; and generation of empirical evidence on key measurement properties of a PRO measure, in Chapter 6. The last chapter of the book, Chapter 7, discusses key issues in the design and planning, implementation (i.e. data collection) and reporting (or use) of PRO assessments in different settings.

The future for PRO measurement is exciting, and the long-held vision of structured systematic PRO measurement becoming 'standard practice' in both clinical research and practice is no longer a far-fetched dream, albeit its full realization would require concerted efforts by researchers and all key stakeholders in the field. For this to move forward requires involvement of patients (those living with a chronic disease) not only as subjects but also as a collaborator/partner in research and practice.

Darmstadt, Germany — Paul Kamudoni
Khon Kaen, Thailand — Nutjaree Johns
Hatfield, UK — Sam S. Salek

Contents

Part I

A New Roadmap for Development of a PRO Measure

1 Overview

The assessment of health outcomes is rapidly evolving, with a growing interest in outcomes reported by the patient. Patient-reported outcomes (PROs) constitute any report of the status of a patient's health condition that comes directly from the patient without any interpretation of the patient's response by a clinician or anyone else (US Food and Drug Administration 2009). Examples include patient's report of their symptoms, physical function or patient satisfaction. However, emphasis on the patients' own self-report has increased in the last two decades.

The current emphasis on PROs is driven by various factors. First, there is a growing recognition of the need to capture patients' perspectives of illness and healthcare interventions, both in routine clinical practice and resource allocation decision-making, to enhance patient centricity. For example, within the drug regulatory context, initiatives to foster 'patient-centred' drug development are underway both at the Food and Drug Administration (FDA) and at the European Medicines Agency (EMA) (Coons et al. 2011; Basch 2013). Second, in Western countries and

---

Living with a Chronic Disease

(Anecdote)

Having a chronic illness, Molly thought, was like being invaded. Her grandmother back in Michigan used to tell about the day one of their cows got loose and wandered into the parlor, and the awful time they had getting her out. That was exactly what Molly's arthritis was like: as if some big old cow had got into her house and wouldn't go away. It just sat there, taking up space in her life and making everything more difficult, mooing loudly from time to time and making cow pies, and all she could do really was edge around it and put up with it.

When other people first became aware of the cow, they expressed concern and anxiety. They suggested strategies for getting the animal out of Molly's parlor: remedies and doctors and procedures, some mainstream and some New Age. They related anecdotes of friends who had removed their own cows in one way or another. But after a while they had exhausted their suggestions. Then they usually began to pretend that the cow wasn't there, and they preferred for Molly to go along with the pretense.

Alison Lurie, The Last Resort

P. Kamudoni et al., *Living with Chronic Disease: Measuring Important Patient-Reported Outcomes*, https://doi.org/10.1007/978-981-10-8414-0_1

more recently in emerging economies, chronic, non-communicable and lifestyle diseases account for an increasing share of disease burden (World Health Organisation 2014). Longterm conditions such as cancer, diabetes, Alzheimer and cardiovascular disease, are a growing health challenge. In chronic diseases, maintaining a comfortable, functional and satisfying life, rather than complete cure from disease, is an important goal of therapy (Salek and Luscombe 1992). Further, improvements in medical care and general living conditions have meant that people are now living longer, leading to an increase in conditions related to aging, such as dementia and Parkinson's disease. This has led to a shift in the focus from increasing life expectancy towards improvement of functional ability and quality of life. Finally, PROs constitute outcomes of high importance to patients. Generally, patients with long-term conditions (LTCs) are concerned with symptoms they experience on a day-to-day basis and the overall quality of their life as well as how these might be affected by potential treatments. A typical patient may ask 'Can I go out with friends without worrying that I may vomit due to the chemotherapy?' (Lohr and Zebrack 2009). Therefore, questions used in PROs are more relevant outcomes to patients than clinical and laboratory measurements/outcomes.

Patient-Reported Outcome as a Concept

Various outcomes may be assessed based on the information reported by the patients, including symptoms, functioning (activity limitations), health-related quality of life (HRQoL), satisfaction with care or treatment, treatment experience, work productivity impairment and adherence to treatment (Table 1.1). The relevance and importance of the different PRO concepts depend on the context of use and objectives of assessment. In clinical research, symptoms and functional impairment, core to a disease, may be of most interest. For example, the FDA's office of Hematology and Oncology Products has suggested consideration of three PRO concepts in cancer trials—symptomatic adverse events, physical functioning and disease-related symptoms (Kluetz et al. 2016). The US National Cancer Institute's Symptom Management and Health Related Quality of Life Steering Committee recently developed a core symptom set to be assessed across oncology trials, based on a systematic literature review and expert consensus (Reeve et al. 2014). Twelve symptoms including fatigue, insomnia, pain and anorexia (appetite loss) have been recommended (Reeve et al. 2014). Other concepts, which may be distal/indirect to the disease, such as work productivity/disability, may be of particular interest in other contexts of use e.g. during health technology assessment.

Scope for the Use of PROs

PROs have been employed in medicines development programmes since the 1970s/1980s, for example in programmes involving analgesics and other CNS indications. Nevertheless, there has been a marked increase in their use over the last two decades. This has encouraged the issuance of guidelines by drug regulatory agencies

Table 1.1 Patient-reported outcome concept

PRO concept	Description
Symptom	Symptoms are proximal to the disease or its treatment and cover impairment of psychological, physiological or anatomical structure or function (Doward et al. 2010)
Functional ability/activity limitation	Disability in performance of activities in the manner considered normal for a specific age group (Doward et al. 2010; McKenna 2011) and includes domains such as activities of daily living and social functioning
HRQoL	The overall functional effect of an illness as well as therapy as perceived by the patients (Padilla et al. 1996). As a multidimensional concept, HRQoL includes symptoms and functional status domains as well as patient's perception of their health status
QoL	From a needs-based perspective, this represents the degree to which patients' needs are met, irrespective of functional ability (McKenna 2011)
Satisfaction with care	Assesses acceptability of the process of care (e.g. aspects of treatment) to the patients
Patient preference information	Qualitative or quantitative assessments of the relative desirability/acceptability to patients of specified alternatives or choices among attributes (e.g. drug's benefits and risks) that differ among alternative interventions[a]
Work productivity	The ability to work and perform regular work activities

[a]http://www.fda.gov/downloads/medicaldevices/deviceregulationandguidance/guidancedocuments/ucm446680.pdf

such as the US FDA and EMA on the use of PROs during market authorization application of new medicines. HRQoL and other PRO data appeared in the scientific discussions of 34% of products submitted between 1995 and 2005 (Bottomley et al. 2009). Gnanasakthy et al. (2013) observed that out of the 308 new molecular entities (NMEs) and biologics license applications (BLAs) granted approval by the US FDA between 2000 and 2012, PRO claims were approved in 70 (23%), with the PROs being the primary endpoint in the majority (81%) of the cases.

Within drug regulatory settings, different national agencies have different views. The FDA has shown tendencies towards more proximal outcomes such as symptoms and functioning, relative to distal outcomes such as HRQoL. On the other hand, the EMA has a particular interest in HRQoL and encourages its inclusion as an endpoint in clinical trials. Over the period 2010–2014, the FDA granted labels for various PRO concepts in oncology including improvement in pain related to prostate cancer (based on Brief Pain Inventory, Short Form), improvement of symptoms associated with myelofibrosis (based on Myelofibrosis Symptom Assessment Form) and visual disturbances (based on Visual Symptom Assessment Questionnaire, anaplastic lymphoma kinase) (Gnanasakthy et al. 2016).

Use of PROs has also been extended to other contexts, such as clinical practice, for example, the monitoring of impacts of disease and its treatment, screening of patients experiencing major side effects and during multidisciplinary team meetings/discussions (Greenhalgh 2009). There are now efforts across various healthcare systems to use patient-reported outcome measures (PROMs) for monitoring the performance of the healthcare system, not only in the UK but also in other countries such as Sweden and the USA. In Sweden, disease-specific clinical databases (quality registers) have been established under the watch of the medical profession and in the USA; this has covered spinal conditions in New England and for primary care in Pittsburgh (Black 2013). In the English NHS, since 2009, all healthcare providers treating NHS patients for hip or knee replacement, groin hernia repair and varicose vein surgery have been required to assess PROs before and after treatment involving 485,000 patients (Devlin and Appleby 2010). This highlights the pace and scope of the use of PROs.

Assessing PROs in Long-Term Conditions

Maintaining a normal and productive life (encompassing physical, mental and social well-being) is an important, if not the ultimate, goal of treatment for individuals with LTCs. Thus, capturing the experience and perspective of the patient in relation to their condition/health is an essential element of the clinical management of LTC. For example, enhancing the quality of life (QoL) of people living with LTCs is the second domain of the NHS Outcomes Framework for England and Wales—a set of indicators for assessing the performance of the NHS in England and Wales (Department of Health 2014). Five domains of HRQoL based on the EQ-5D are employed as indicators for the domain, including mobility, self-care activities, pain or discomfort, feeling anxious or depressed.

We illustrate the role of PROs in chronic illnesses using SLE as an example. SLE is a chronic autoimmune disease that affects multiple body systems and is most prevalent among women of child-bearing age (the female to male ratio of prevalence is 9:1) (Lisnevskaia et al. 2014). Clinical manifestations in early disease stages (~first 5 years) include discoid lesions, arthritis, serositis, psychosis or seizures (Bertsias et al. 2008). In addition, various comorbidities are common, including infections, atherosclerosis, hypertension and lupus nephritis. Over the course of the disease, patients accumulate damage across various body systems/organs such as osteonecrosis and cataracts associated with long-term use of corticosteroid therapy, cardiovascular and neuropsychiatric damage and musculoskeletal damage (Gladman et al. 2003). Thus impacts on daily life and QoL are driven by multiple factors including disease activity, complications of disease, treatment side effects as well as overall cumulative damage.

Patients with SLE are most concerned about signs and symptoms such as joint pain, fatigue, skin manifestations—malar, facial or body rash—skin sensitivity and alopecia (Robinson and Aguilar 2010). The pain and stiffness in the joints have been described as unpredictable, disabling and incapacitating, and patients have reported feeling frustrated and a sense of being incapable of performing tasks as a result of their fatigue (Robinson and Aguilar 2010). One patient described their experience of pain in the following way:

> *Joint pain stops me walking very far. I used to go to the gym, I don't now. I used to swim quite a lot, I don't do that now. My knees sometimes give way. My leg gives way so I am a bit frightened of actually coming out of the changing rooms, you know on to the side of the pool and the results of that, of not doing those things have made me gain so much weight and I have put so much on I feel like it has hampered my joints and it is like a vicious circle that I don't know how to break* (Robinson and Aguilar 2010).

Life impacts of greatest concern to SLE patients have included impacts on work life, recreation, social life and emotional well-being; for example, patients have reported feeling a low sense of self-esteem and impaired self-image as a result of skin manifestations (e.g. malar rash) and side effects of treatment such as weight gain (Sutanto et al. 2013). One patient described their situation as follows:

> *Embarrassment, definitely, because of the scarring. It's really awful and some people … I don't think they mean to, but, 'what is that?', 'what is that on your face?', or 'what happened to you?', and it's a little frustrating having to explain, you don't feel like it* (Robinson and Aguilar 2010).

Due to the complexity of SLE, any single outcome domain such as disease activity or cumulative damage may not accurately represent the patient's health status. Therefore, experiential evidence—based on patient's perspective of symptoms and QoL covering the totality of the different consequences of the condition—is essential to accurately assess health status. Even more critically, a holistic understanding of disease outcomes is crucial in making benefit-risk assessment for the individual patient. This means PROs may play a vital role alongside other types of information considered in the clinical management of SLE.

In chronic skin conditions such as rosacea and acne, the perspective of the patients may provide valuable information about disease severity, given the scarcity of appropriate and meaningful disease activity measures or biomarkers (Grob 2007; Wörle et al. 2007). In such cases, patient-reported symptoms and daily life impacts could be a plausible predictor/proxy for disease activity. For example, in hyperhidrosis, the Hyperhidrosis Disease Severity Score (HDSS), recommended for measuring severity of hyperhidrosis in various disease clinical guidelines, assesses the severity of hyperhidrosis based on interference in everyday life.

Clinicians may omit assessment of PROs such as daily life impacts thinking that these may be deduced from clinical observation or biomedical parameters. Empirical evidence suggests that PRO concepts such as 'HRQoL' and symptoms are unique from disease severity, although there may be some linkages (Schmitt and Ford 2007). It may not be possible to accurately infer one from the other. Patients may experience great impairment even with low disease severity and vice versa; patients may have high disease severity and yet experience minimal life impairment (Basra and Shahrukh 2009). Clinical assessments may not always agree with patients' own assessment of their own health status (Jemec and Wulf 1996; Hermansen et al. 2002). Moreover, patients' satisfaction with care has been reported to be linked to the magnitude of HRQoL impairment and less to severity of disease (Renzi et al. 2001). This highlights the importance of PROs as a key health outcome in their own right.

The usefulness of PRO assessment in LTCs may be summarised as follows:

- *Monitoring outcomes.* PROs may support the identification of underdiagnosed and unrecognised health issues.
- *Facilitating the patient—clinician communication and shared decision-making.* PRO assessment may legitimise or facilitate discussion about daily life issues such as psychosocial issues with clinicians. Information on patient experience and preferences related to treatments and health outcomes may be discussed between patients and clinicians to decide on treatment strategy.
- *Supporting patient self-management.* PRO assessment may adjust patient's expectations from treatment for their condition. Patients can use PRO measure to track changes in their condition, and this, if linked to patient's electronic health record, could be of benefit to other services involved in providing care for the patient.
- *Framework for risk-benefit assessment.* PROs such as HRQoL, which capture the patient's own evaluation of their overall health, typically considering multiple domains provide a robust framework for benefit-risk assessment of medicines, as well as communication of such information to the patient. For example, where therapy is successful in eliminating the primary symptoms associated with a condition but results in other limitations in patient's life.

Further, inclusion of PRO assessments in clinical studies of LTCs may be useful in a number of ways:

- *Provides a patient perspective on the effectiveness and safety of a medicine.* For medicines with similar effectiveness profiles, for example, similar progression-free survival rate, PRO information such as the patient-reported outcome version of the Common Terminology Criteria for Adverse Events (PRO-CTCAE) may support measurement of the differential impact on patients' well-being influenced by tolerability of the new medicine and its toxicity profile differences.
- *Supports optimisation of clinical development programmes.* In dose titration studies, PROs such as patient satisfaction—with efficacy, tolerability and convenience—may be used in the selection of appropriate doses that offer meaningful outcomes. The patterns of variability in disease-specific PROs may facilitate the identification of key subgroups of patients—patients who benefit the most from treatment.
- *Supports labelling claims.* Clinical trial results on PROs such as symptoms, HRQoL and functional status may be used in product labelling. Such information might be informative to patients as well as clinicians in assessing the benefit-risk balance of individual drugs in the clinic.
- *Supports reimbursement applications.* In addition to clinical outcomes, health authorities and payers are interested in PROs such as HRQoL, because of the emphasis on patient centricity. In addition, HRQoL has a potential being used as an aid to resource allocation decision-making by allowing comparisons across different disease conditions.

Approaches to Measuring PROs

The somewhat abstract nature of PROs, based on patient's subjective perception, requires the use of measurement technique that is robust, possessing the appropriate precision. To ensure the required precision of PRO assessment, the selected measurement approach needs to be fit for the purpose and appropriate for the intended context of use. This entails a choice between different types of instruments such as individualised, disease-specific, domain-specific, therapeutic area specific, or generic (Table 1.2) as well as consideration of the empirical evidence supporting use of the measure. The FDA has published a guidance describing standards for PRO measures used in drug development programmes. In addition, professional societies such as ISOQOL, ISPOR and EADV have proposed their own best practice and recommendations on the use of PROs. The common attributes identified by the aforementioned organisations are summarised below:

- *Conceptual framework and measurement model.* Documentation of description of the concepts assessed by a measure. Empirical evidence supporting the internal structure of the measure needs to be available, reflecting the conceptual framework.
- *Acceptability and practicality.* The ease of completion of an instrument as well as the level of patient burden associated with completing a measure. Similarly, the ease of administering a measure as well as its feasibility in the context of use.
- *Content validity.* Appropriateness of a measure's content for its target population. This is supported by qualitative evidence documenting the involvement of the target patient population.
- *Construct validity*. Evidence demonstrating that the measure assesses its intended concept.
- *Reliability*. The magnitude of measurement errors associated with scores of a PRO measure.

Table 1.2 Classification of PRO measures

Instrument	Description
Individualised	Allows patients to choose the items included in the instrument, as well as indicating how important they are to them (Luckett et al. 2009)
Disease-specific	Intended for assessing PRO concepts in specific patient populations, including content that clinicians and patient consider important for a given condition
Therapeutic area specific	Is a hybrid between disease-specific and generic instruments, with a broader scope than disease-specific instruments, to allow application in more than one disease, while on the other hand, they maintain content that is relevant to the group of diseases beyond generic measures (Salek 1998)
Domain-specific	Assesses a specific function or impact area and is broadly applicable across different patient/healthy populations, e.g. *the PROMIS physical function item bank*
Generic	Assesses general health status/HRQL/QoL and is broadly applicable across different patient/healthy populations, e.g. *Nottingham Health Profile (NHP)*

- *Responsiveness to change.* The ability of scores of a measure to capture any changes in the patient's condition.
- *Interpretability of scores.* Availability of information facilitating the qualitative interpretation of scores of a PRO measure.

It is generally agreed that a robust process underpinning development of PRO measures could ensure the precision of attributes described above. The process of PRO measure development has become complex and lengthy, reflecting the measurement demands which the modern PRO measures must withstand. Patient involvement was virtually non-existent for legacy/early PRO measures, with researchers drafting items based on their own understanding (Nijsten 2012). Only a few psychometric attributes were assessed for such measures; for example, construct validity and reliability, and no further psychometric testing would take place. In contrast, the content of the new generation of PRO measures is based on patient input. Also, in addition to classical psychometric attributes (i.e. reliability, construct validity and responsiveness), attributes such as response category functioning, differential item functioning and internal structure are explored. In summary, the process of developing a new PRO measure involves the following steps:

- Literature review and developing rationale for new instrument.
- Qualitative study to elicit concepts for the measure.
- Item/cognitive interviewing to evaluate the elicited concepts.
- Quantitative study to evaluate the psychometric attributes including classical test theory and modern test theory.

This evolution largely reflects developments in the context and environment in which PROs are developed and used. This will be explored fully in the subsequent chapters with examples illustrating the steps listed above.

Aims and Objectives

It is hoped that this book will provide a roadmap for development and application of patient-reported outcome measures, for use in both clinical research and practice.

The objectives of this book include:

1. To present a unified framework for the development and application of patient-reported outcomes (PROs) consistent with the current generation of PROs.
2. To offer a practical step-by-step guide on the development and application of PROs, based on extensive research in hyperhidrosis.
3. To provide insights into humanistic burden of chronic disease, particularly issues related to their day-to-day life, using hyperhidrosis as a case study.
4. To present a disease model as well as a psychosocial model for chronic disease based on the hyperhidrosis model.

The remaining chapters of the book are as follows:

- *Chapter 2: Approaches to the development and use of PRO measures: a new roadmap.* This chapter will present a unified PRO framework being proposed in this book, including key concepts, processes and issues. The nature and typology of existing patient-reported outcomes will be described. Detailed description of how PROs are used in various contexts and a checklist of key considerations will be provided. This chapter will also present a unified framework on the process of developing a new generation of PROs. This will cover issues related to the process of assembling a research team, including special considerations on patient engagement. The framework will cover the core steps in the process, as well as the study designs that can be utilised for each step. The framework will demonstrate novelty in terms of inclusion of comprehensive qualitative research, integration of conventional (i.e. classical test theory) and modern (i.e. modern test theory) test approaches in PRO development/validation work, use of new channels of patient recruitment and gathering of data, multiple ways of involving patients in the development of PROs such patient engagement and integrating new technologies such as smart phones in PRO use or measurement.
- *Chapter 3: Conceptualisation and qualitative development of a PRO measure.* The purpose of this chapter and the subsequent three chapters is to present a case study, illustrating how the framework developed in Chapter 2 may be implemented, step by step. The chapter provides a background on hyperhidrosis (our selected chronic disease for the case study), presenting a disease model, as well as a socioeconomic model reflecting the impacts of hyperhidrosis. In addition, the latter part of the chapter will present further evidence of the impact of hyperhidrosis on the daily life and quality of life of patients, based on qualitative research.
- *Chapter 4: Content validation by Patients and Experts: Is the PRO measure fit for purpose?* This chapter will describe the process of verifying that the content of the patient-reported outcome measure is comprehensive and relevant for intended use. Specifically, the process of involving therapeutic experts and practical ways of engaging patients will be discussed. The processes/strategy described is illustrated using the research carried out in the development of the Hyperhidrosis Quality of Life Index.
- Chapter 5: *Applying modern test theory methods in PRO measure development: Rasch modelling.* The purpose of this chapter is to present alternative ways of refining a patient-reported outcome measures, as well as gaining insights about its internal structure, the functioning of the response categorisation and how well the measure functions across different groups. Specifically, we present an approach based on item response theory. The technique of implementing either approaches is described in detail. Recommendations on how to address friction between approaches are presented. A new checklist supporting the practical implementation of recommendations will be presented.
- *Chapter 6: Assessing the performance of PRO measures against expectations: Psychometric evaluation.* This chapter is intended to present a detailed descrip-

tion of the core/conventional metrics/attributes of patient-reported outcome measures including how free PROs are from error during usage (reliability), how well they function as expected (construct validity), how well they capture relevant changes in patient's condition (responsiveness) and the criteria for interpreting scores. The process of assessing each of the properties is described in detail including the relevant/appropriate study designs. The material is presented using results from the research to develop and assess the Hyperhidrosis Quality of Life Index.

- *Chapter 7: Integrating PRO assessment in clinical trials, routine clinical practice and medicines development programmes.* The purpose of this chapter is to discuss some of the key pitfalls and major issues in the application of patient-reported outcomes in two context of use—routine clinical practice and medicine development programmes. Insights into the opportunities and challenges presented by recent contextual and methodological developments such as the rise in the use of smart phones, collaborative PRO development and interpretability of scores will be elucidated. Recommendations on how these might be addressed are presented. The significance of the unified framework presented and illustrated in the book is also discussed.

References

Basch E (2013) Toward patient-centered drug development in oncology. N Engl J Med 369(5):397–400

Basra MKA, Shahrukh M (2009) Burden of skin diseases. Expert Rev Pharmacoecon Outcomes Res 9(3):271–283

Bertsias G et al (2008) EULAR recommendations for the management of systemic lupus erythematosus. Report of a Task Force of the EULAR Standing Committee for International Clinical Studies Including Therapeutics. Ann Rheum Dis 67(2):195–205

Black N (2013) Patient reported outcome measures could help transform healthcare. BMJ 346:f167

Bottomley A et al (2009) Patient-reported outcomes: assessment and current perspectives of the guidelines of the Food and Drug Administration and the reflection paper of the European Medicines Agency. Eur J Cancer 45(3):347–353

Coons SJ et al (2011) The patient-reported outcome (PRO) consortium: filling measurement gaps for PRO end points to support labeling claims. Clin Pharmacol Ther 90(5):743–748

Department of Health (2014) Title: the NHS outcomes framework 2015/16. Department of Health, London, pp 1–22

Devlin NJ, Appleby J (2010) Getting the most out of PROMS. The Kings Fund, Office of Health Economics, London

Doward LC et al (2010) Patient reported outcomes: looking beyond the label claim. Health Qual Life Outcomes 8:89

Gladman DD et al (2003) Accrual of organ damage over time in patients with systemic lupus erythematosus. J Rheumatol 30(9):1955–1959

Gnanasakthy A et al (2013) Potential of patient-reported outcomes as nonprimary endpoints in clinical trials. Health Qual Life Outcomes 11(1):83

Gnanasakthy A et al (2016) Patient-reported outcomes labeling for products approved by the office of hematology and oncology products of the US Food and Drug Administration (2010–2014). J Clin Oncol 34(16):1928–1934

Greenhalgh J (2009) The applications of PROs in clinical practice: what are they, do they work, and why? Qual Life Res 18(1):115–123
Grob JJ (2007) Why are quality of life instruments not recognized as reference measures in therapeutic trials of chronic skin disorders? J Investig Dermatol 127(10):2299–2301
Hermansen SE et al (2002) Patients' and doctors' assessment of skin disease handicap. Clin Exp Dermatol 27(3):249–250
Jemec GB, Wulf HC (1996) Patient-physician consensus on quality of life in dermatology. Clin Exp Dermatol 21(3):177–179
Kluetz PG et al (2016) Focusing on core patient-reported outcomes in cancer clinical trials: symptomatic adverse events, physical function, and disease-related symptoms. Clin Cancer Res 22(7):1553–1558
Lisnevskaia L et al (2014) Systemic lupus erythematosus. Lancet 384(9957):1878–1888
Lohr KN, Zebrack BJ (2009) Using patient-reported outcomes in clinical practice: challenges and opportunities. Qual Life Res 18(1):99–107
Luckett T et al (2009) Improving patient outcomes through the routine use of patient-reported data in cancer clinics: future directions. Psychooncology 18(11):1129–1138
McKenna SP (2011) Measuring patient-reported outcomes: moving beyond misplaced common sense to hard science. BMC Med 9(1):86
Nijsten T (2012) Dermatology Life Quality Index: time to move forward. J Investig Dermatol 132(1):11–13
Padilla GV et al (1996) Quality of life - cancer. In: Spilker B (ed) Quality of life and pharmacoeconomics in clinical trials, 2nd edn. Lippincott-Raven, Philadelphia, pp 301–308
Reeve BB et al (2014) Recommended patient-reported core set of symptoms to measure in adult cancer treatment trials. J Natl Cancer Inst 106(7):pii: dju129
Renzi C et al (2001) Factors associated with patient satisfaction with care among dermatological outpatients. Br J Dermatol 145(4):617–623
Robinson D, Aguilar D (2010) Impact of systemic lupus erythematosus on health, family, and work: the patient perspective. Arthritis care Res 62(2):266–273
Salek M (1998) Compendium of quality of life instruments. Euromed Communications, Haslemere
Salek MS, Luscombe DK (1992) Health-related quality of life assessment: a review. J Drug Dev 5(3):137–153
Schmitt J, Ford DE (2007) Understanding the relationship between objective disease severity, psoriatic symptoms, illness-related stress, health-related quality of life and depressive symptoms in patients with psoriasis – a structural equations modeling approach. Gen Hosp Psychiatry 29(2):134–140
Sutanto B et al (2013) Experiences and perspectives of adults living with systemic lupus erythematosus: thematic synthesis of qualitative studies. Arthritis Care Res 65(11):1752–1765
US Food and Drug Administration (2009) Guidance for Industry: Patient-reported outcome measures: use in medicinal product development to support labeling claims. Health Qual Life Outcomes 4:79
World Health Organisation (2014) Global health estimates 2014 summary tables: DALY by cause, age and sex, by WHO Regio, 2000–2012. World Health Organisation, Geneva
Wörle B et al (2007) Definition and treatment of primary hyperhidrosis. J German Soc Dermatol 5(7):625–628

Approaches to the Development and Use of PRO Measures: A New Roadmap

2

Various recent developments are driving an evolution in the way PRO measures are developed. For example, drug regulatory agencies (e.g. the FDA) can now be more substantively involved in PRO measure development work; the patients' role is now seen as going beyond being a study subject to being involved as research partners. Use of modern test theory in development of scoring algorithms and overall measure development work is now the new 'gold standard'.

This is a watershed moment in the field of PRO measurement; there is now an opportunity to build on the many various developments to create a unified framework and a streamlined roadmap for PRO measure development. Such new framework would aim to enhance hypotheses-driven measure validation, greater use of mixed research methods, i.e. a stronger integration between qualitative and quantitative methods, taking full advantage of the capabilities within modern test theory and consensus on generalisability of PRO measurement metrics.

This book sets out to propose a framework for PRO measure development, reflecting the issues highlighted above, to further streamline the measure development process. The steps proposed in the framework are applicable to most PROs; a

---

The challenge

(anecdote)

In the measurement of glucose, the glucose assay and computational algorithm are embodied in the instrument that is used to provide glucose readings…The quality of life measurement process is essentially an assay that defines the construct, uses question and response formats to obtain answers, and has an algorithm that scores those responses to yield quality of life readings. However, because of the subjectivity and indirect measurement issues, it is harder to adopt a standard assay for quality of life.

Testa 2000

P. Kamudoni et al., *Living with Chronic Disease: Measuring Important Patient-Reported Outcomes*, https://doi.org/10.1007/978-981-10-8414-0_2

multidimensional health-related quality of life (HRQoL) addressing complexities and key challenges has been illustrated in the case studies presented in the book.

Traditionally, PRO instruments have been classified as individualised, disease-specific, therapeutic area-specific, domain-specific and generic, as described in greater detail in Chap. 1. The Emergence of domain-specific measures as well as application of common metrics for assessing concepts, based on item response theory (IRT) and item banking, has made the traditional delineation of measures less relevant. Otherwise, the choice of appropriate measure(s) for a specific context depends on the objectives of data collection, the environment of the application and methodological and practical considerations (Patrick and Deyo 1989). Often, the different measure types may be combined in a single study or PRO data collection exercise, to address multiple objectives.

Characteristics of a PROM: Core Measurement Attributes

There is strong consensus among regulatory authorities such as the FDA and the EMA as well as professional agencies such as the International Society of Quality of Life Research (ISOQOL) regarding core attributes required to support a measure's credibility within a given context of use. This includes qualitative as well as quantitative (measurement) attributes. The latter are largely based on classical techniques and theories applied in psychological measurement, which assumes existence of a true score reflecting the underlying concept of interest, where the goal of measurement is to minimise measurement error in estimating the true score. They are described in detail below.

Conceptual Framework

A conceptual framework outlines the concepts intended to be measured, the rationale for their measurement and how the domains relate to other concepts (Lohr 2002; Food and Drug Administration 2009). Interrelationships between concept, domains and items are ideally depicted graphically. Please see Fig. 3.1, for an illustration. The conceptual framework evolves throughout PROM development; early versions are considered hypothetical and are based on literature review and input from clinical experts, while later versions are based on fieldwork qualitative research. This document serves as a blueprint for the instrument, including the internal scaling structure and measurement model (Rothman et al. 2007). The process of developing a conceptual framework not only ensures that the purported constructs are appropriately measured but also facilitates the interpretation of the data.

Measurement Models and Scoring Algorithms

The measurement model (or scale and subscale structure) of a PRO measure translates the conceptual framework of the PROM into measurable scores and has implications for the definition of the underlying target concept and any inferential use of the PROM. For instance, items forming a subscale are assumed to be homogenous and to address similar aspects of a concept, while simple summation of items into a single scale score assumes that the items are weighted equally and are assessing a single underlying concept (Fayers and Machin 2007). In contrast, the weighting approach assigns a mathematical score to individual items, according to relative severity of each item within the construct, which may be theoretical or empirically based (Streiner and Norman 2008). The rationale and evidence underpinning proposed scaling structures and scoring algorithms form a core part of validity evidence.

Acceptability and Practicality

Acceptability of an instrument by the final users (e.g. patients) has a bearing on not only respondents' motivation to complete the questionnaire but also on the integrity of the data obtained. The instrument must be easy to complete, imposing the least burden on the respondents (Both et al. 2007). For instance, the measure should not be unnecessarily lengthy and must be well organised, allowing for easy navigation and completion. Loss of spontaneity to the response process as the respondents become fatigued may lead to avoidable errors or undesirable response behaviours, for example, 'satisficing' (Streiner and Norman 2008).

On the other hand, the effort required to administer the instrument and collect and process data must be minimal to make the use of the instrument (Salek 1998). This is a particularly important consideration in routine clinical practice. If data collection and processing are excessively burdensome, avoidable errors may creep in during the process as the administrators become less careful.

Validity

As most PRO concepts such as HRQoL tend to be unobservable and abstract, evidence that an instrument assesses what is intended, demonstrating validity of the measurements, is important (Fayers and Machin 2007). A lack of such evidence may risk misleading inferences, as there would be no certainty regarding what actually is being measured (Haynes et al. 1995). Thus, the validity attribute relates to a particular use of scales and is not an inherent trait of the instrument (Messick 1988). As such, PROM validation is an ongoing process of generating evidence supporting various inferences based on the instrument (Streiner and Norman 2008). Validity is often described in terms of three different forms including content validity, which relates to the appropriateness of the content; construct validity, which covers the quantitative data supporting particular use of the measure; and criterion validity, which demonstrates consistency between a measure and a gold standard.

Content Validity

The appropriateness of a PRO measure's content vis-a-vis targeted concepts and intended settings of use is core to a measure's overall validity and has implications for other measurement properties. Content validity relates to the adequacy or comprehensiveness of the items, domains and other elements of the instrument in reflecting/covering the underlying concept(s) being measured (Salek 1998; Patrick et al. 2011b).

Different types of information contribute to content validity evidence including (1) a clear conceptual framework, as a basis for the instrument; (2) a well-documented, organised and structured process of content development (Terwee et al. 2007), allowing the tracking of items and other elements to their source; and (3) qualitative research capturing target population's perspective on the concepts of interest (how they experience, understand and discuss the concepts) (Patrick et al. 2011b). Further sources of information worth considering include item distribution statistics showing frequency of endorsement of items, as well as ceiling or floor effects (proportion of patients on choosing the extreme options), and data on how well the items cover different levels of a concept, for example, based on item distribution maps from item response theory analyses.

Although a dedicated test for content validity is not available, expert ratings as well as qualitative feedback are often used (Streiner and Norman 2008). A structured and rigorous approach is usually followed in the collection and analysis of data (e.g. DELPHI panels). Quite often content validity is confused with face validity. The latter relates to the acceptance conferred by lay persons that the instrument appears to be sound and relevant (Lynn 1986). The assessment of face validity is based on perception and there is no rigorous assessment or quantification (Lynn 1986; Frost et al. 2007a, b).

Construct Validity

PRO concepts suffer from lack of a dedicated statistical proof for their existence. Thus, interpretation of PRO measure scores is rather theoretical and hypothetical and rests on the evidence supporting theoretical hypothesis, to warrant inferences being made on the scores (Terwee et al. 2007). Such evidence represents the construct validity of a measure.

Studies for demonstrating construct validity vary in design, although they all have common footing on defining and testing different hypothesis related to the underlying construct. Common study designs for construct validity are presented below. A unified view of validity considers all forms of validity as being subsumed under construct validity based on the argument that construct interpretation undergirds all score-based inferences; thus, the various forms of validity are indeed only supporting that the construct is valid (Messick 1988).

Known groups or discriminant validity—involves testing hypothesis relating to group differences in scores of patient, anticipated to differ. Such groups are usually based on some important clinical variable, for instance, level of disease severity or the localisation of the sweating, in the case of hyperhidrosis.

Convergent and divergent validity—is based on expected relationships between a scale and other measures assessing a similar construct. A scale is expected to show high correlation (convergence) with other scales assessing similar constructs, and conversely a low correlation (divergence) would be expected with other measures (scales) assessing unrelated constructs (Streiner and Norman 2008).

Criterion Validity

Criterion validity assesses the extent to which a measure agrees with an external gold standard measure and how well the new measure is consistent with and captures the essence of the gold standard (Frost et al. 2007a). This includes situations where the gold standard is measured at the same time as the new measure, reflecting *concurrent criterion validity* as well as where the gold standard is only observed at a later date, *predictive criterion validity.* For most PRO concepts, measures with proven validity serving as gold standards are not available; thus, criterion validity may have little relevance in the context of most PRO measurement (Salek and Luscombe 1992). Indeed, existence of such gold standards would obviate need to develop PRO measures.

Reliability

In the context of classical test theory (CTT), reliability is conceptualised as the degree to which scores of an instrument reflect the true score (a hypothetical score thought to be representing the underlying condition) (Nunnally and Bernstein 1994). In other words, this is the proportion of total variance in measurement accounted for by true score after measurement error is accounted for (Streiner and Norman 2008), i.e. the signal-to-noise ratio (Guyatt et al. 1993). The relationship between reliability and other measurement attributes, e.g. validity and responsiveness, is a widely discussed topic. While reliability is clearly a distinct attribute, it may be challenging to demonstrate responsiveness or be able to discriminate between different groups, if a measure lacks reliability.

Reliability has practical implications on the design of studies employing a PROM (Streiner and Norman 2008). For example, in clinical trials, reliability is conversely related to power and sample sizes, i.e. a less reliable PROM may require a larger sample to show a particular effect size relative to a more reliable measure.

Reliability relates to both the consistency and reproducibility of scores from an instrument and can be determined in different ways.

Internal Consistency

Internal consistency looks at 'homogeneity' among items belonging to a single scale or domain, whether the items are tapping into the underlying construct equally strongly (Fayers and Machin 2007). The assumption made here is that as items in a single scale are meant to be assessing different aspects of the same underlying construct, the items are interrelated through their relationship with this construct. Internal consistency, therefore, captures the proportion of scale score total variance attributable to a common source among the items (DeVellis 2016).

Split-Half Reliability

Split-half reliability looks at a scale's consistency by evaluating the inter-correlation between two halves of a scale (Streiner and Norman 2008). The many possibilities for creating the two halves can be challenging, and the following common approaches are used: first half-second half split, odd-even items and balanced based on external criteria to divide the scale in different ways. Correlating one half of the scale to the other implies that the correlation represents reliability of a single half of the scale, to obtain the reliability of the entire scale the Spearman-Brown formula has to be applied (DeVellis 2016).

Inter-Rater Reliability

Inter-rater reliability assesses the level of agreement in ratings on subjects made by different judges, following two alternative approaches: 'consistency' or 'absolute agreement'. Inter-rater consistency relates to the amount of proportion that deviates from means as different experts rate an item while absolute agreement constitutes the exact agreement in the ratings made by different judges (Wynd et al. 2003). This form of reliability is of particular importance in observer- or interviewer-administered instruments (Salek 1998).

Temporal Stability (Test-Retest Reliability)

Temporal stability assesses the reproducibility of scores over time. It is expected that if the instrument is used in patients whose condition has not changed, the scores obtained on the two assessments should be similar. As the underlying construct will not have changed, the correlation of the two assessments gives the degree to which the measured concept actually determines the observed scores (DeVellis 2016).

Responsiveness

The capability of a PRO measure to capture important changes in concepts of interest, for example, specific patient symptoms, is a requirement for the longitudinal application of PRO measure (Epstein 2000). Responsiveness captures a notion of the ability to capture (minimal) changes considered important by the patient, in addition to statistical significance, i.e. any score changes beyond chance (Revicki et al. 2008).

Given the intent to identify true changes over and above inter-temporal variability in the scores, reliability is necessary to responsiveness (Streiner and Norman 2008). Testing a PRO measure for responsiveness requires a longitudinal study design, where hypotheses relating to magnitude of change relative to external criteria are tested.

The controversial issues related to responsiveness include whether responsiveness should be considered as a separate attribute unique from validity or reliability (Guyatt et al. 1987) or whether it is part and parcel of an instrument's validity (Hays and Hadorn 1992; Liang 2000). Others use the term 'longitudinal validity' to ensure separation of issues related to sensitivity to change from whether that change is indeed credible.

Given the interdependencies and the practicality of assessing responsiveness vis-a-vis longitudinal validity, such demarcation is blurred and of little practical significance.

Interpretability

Given the abstract nature of PRO concepts, scores often lack an intrinsic qualitative meaning. Thus, information supporting their meaningful interpretation is an important part of a measure's key attributes. Further, statistical significance, i.e. indicating an effect beyond chance, is not informative on clinical relevance of significance of observed magnitude of effect. Clinical significance criterion is consistent with the amount of change in the score that is large enough to require a change in treatment (Wyrwich et al. 2005).

Various types of information may be generated to support interpretation of absolute scores as well as change scores. Score categorisation (scale banding systems), normative values and mapping algorithms are useful for classifying patients based on absolute scores, while minimal clinically important difference (MCID) is relevant for interpreting change scores.

Characteristics of a PROM: Additional Attributes

Response Scales

The scaling employed for capturing item responses plays a key role in how well the concept being addressed by an instrument's item is assessed. The appropriateness of the choice of scale (e.g. *visual analogue scales (VAS), rating scales, Likert, adjectival scale*) may depend on the study aims, the nature of the disease condition and its treatment, the concept being measured, the mode of administration and target population (Patrick et al. 2011a). VAS and rating scales offer a continuous continuum and hence may be more suitable for symptoms such as pain. On the other hand, adjectival and Likert scales are ordinal and might be more appropriate for assessing variables like frequency or intensity of daily life impacts. While VAS seems more sensitive, the available finesse offered by the continuous nature of the scale is beyond the human capability to detect or distinguish small changes, such that this may introduce noise in the process (Streiner and Norman 2008).

When choosing a scale for a measurement instrument, one is faced with finding the balance between the desirable precision of the measure and factors such as spontaneity, target population, practicality and useful friendliness. The number of response categories and the adjectives used as response option indicators influence respondent's comprehension and consistency of responses. Among fully labelled scales, polar-point labelled scales and number-based ranking, labelled scales had the highest number of extreme positives (Dillman 2007).

Frame of Reference

Frame of reference, which is also referred to as 'recall period', needs to be specified for an instrument reflecting the period of time respondents are to consider in providing their responses. As longer periods, for instance, exceeding 1 month, are associated with greater recall bias (Frost et al. 2007a), the shortest recall period feasible is always preferred. Norquist et al. (2011) proposed criteria for judging the appropriateness of a recall period, where the construct being measured; its time course; the purpose for measurement, for instance, assessing treatment benefit in clinical trials; and the target patient population and burden on respondents. For example, acute symptoms that show rapid fluctuation such as pain may best be assessed with a shorter time frame, such as 'at present', while concepts related to psychosocial functioning or activities of daily living may not show much fluctuation on day-to-day basis and thus may optimally be assessed with a weekly to monthly recall period (Frost et al. 2007a). Choice of recall, therefore, needs to be appropriate for the condition and the timing of assessment, while imposing minimal burden on the patient (Kerr et al. 2010).

Mode of Administration

The deployment of a PRO measure during data collection has implications on psychometric attributes; as well as the final data collected. As such, validity evidence is considered specific to each data collection mode (Dalal et al. 2011). Mixing of PRO data collected using different modes is not recommended during clinical trials, as the observed effect size may be attenuated, unless equivalence of the modes is demonstrated (Coons et al. 2009). The appropriateness of a mode depends on the purpose of PRO assessment, target population, their reading and writing abilities, the aims of the study, the characteristics of the disease condition and its treatment, the particular construct being assessed and the recall period (Patrick et al. 2011a).

PRO measures may be deployed in different formats, including (1) interview format, (2) paper-and-pencil self-completion, (3) electronic PRO self-completion and (4) interactive voice response system. The delivery setting may also be different, such as 'in person' at study centre or in subject's own environment such as 'at home'.

Interview Format

This involves a trained interviewer reading out items of a PRO measure to a study participant and subsequently noting down responses. Key advantages include the ability to verify who is actually responding to the PRO measure and the opportunity for respondents to ask questions where they do not understand, which may result in better compliance (Salek and Luscombe 1992).

Paper-and-Pencil Self-Completion

This remains one of the most frequently used deployment approaches and involves asking respondents to complete a paper form of the PRO measure. The PRO measures may be delivered 'in-person', such as in the clinic, where a member of the research team is available during the completion process, to provide instructions and respond to any questions that may come up (Salek and Luscombe 1992). Alternatively, data collection may be done via post or other ways, making it possible for respondents to complete PRO measures in their own environment.

Electronic PRO (ePRO) Self-Completion

The widespread adoption of computing devices and the Internet have made it possible to program PRO measures into electronic format and to easily deploy this for data collection. The measures can be delivered via (1) a dedicated device where the programmed ePRO is loaded; (2) a webpage, for online completion, for example, through a dedicated Internet portal; or (3) subject's own mobile devices where the ePRO measure is loaded; this is known as 'bring your own device' approach.

The ePRO format offers a number of advantages, including (1) lack of geographical restriction to data collection, i.e. capability to hard-to-reach populations (Tweet et al. 2011); (2) additional aspects facilitating completion which are programmable into the ePRO format such as complex skip patterns, input data validation rules and reminders provide opportunity to reduce error rates and respondent burden (Dillman 2007); and (3) automation of certain secondary data processing and management tasks further reducing administrative burden and error rates.

Interactive Voice Response (IVR) Self-Completion

A variant of the electronic format is where the PRO measures are deployed via telephone or other devices using interactive voice response (IVR) system. Instructions, items and response options are voice-read to subjects, and responses can be provided by voice or by keying in numbers on a keypad (in the case of telephone).

Recent developments in voice technology and machine learning have opened up new possibilities for designing IVR systems, e.g. eliminating the tedious aspects of IVR such as repetitively asking respondents to spell out letters. This is an area of great potential for improving patient (or subject) centricity of PRO assessment.

A Roadmap for the Development of a PROM

Although consensus on standards related to attributes has allowed greater alignment on study designs for generating the required validity evidence, the increasing complexity of the process, brought about by recent methodological advances, new roles assumed by stakeholders (regulators; patients), new models for doing PROM development work and demanding contexts in which PRO measures are being deployed, calls for a rethinking of the measure development process. We propose a unified roadmap for PROM development, to further streamline the process (Fig. 2.1).

Roadmap steps	Patient engagement: patient input into research process	Consultation with key stakeholders (e.g. patients, clinicians, regulatory agencies)	Innovative approaches initiatives
Step 1. Define objectives of development of the PRO measure	▪ Determine the need for a new PRO measure ▪ Frame goals and scope of a PRO measure development.	▪ Discuss the need and potential utility (positioning) of the new PRO measure, and broad research approach.	Collaborate or partner with relevant patient groups and other stakeholders on PRO measure development programme
Step 2. Generate hypothesis and conceptualise the PRO measure: disease model/hypothetical conceptual physico-phsychosocial model	▪ Consult relevant qualitative literature ▪ Define core concept, and identify relevant domains relevant qualitative literature	▪ Review disease/conceptual models ▪ Review study plans and protocols.	Analyse publicly accessible relevant social media information (within the confines of research ethics) Use mixed methods for conceptual development (e.g. group concept mapping with stakeholders)
Step 3. Gather and select item concepts: concept elicitation/ qualitative research	▪ Input into study design (e.g. eligibility criteria) ▪ Support study participant recruitment ▪ Participate in data collection (e.g. interviews) Support qualitative data analysis, validation of qualitative transcripts and interpretation process (i.e. data coding).	▪ Feedback on qualitative research study design (e.g. target population, topic guide).	Utilise existing item banks as a source of items for targeted themes / subdomains.
Step 4. Design and build the PRO measure: content definition/item generation	▪ Prioritisation of themes ▪ Crafting of items, response options and other content elements (i.e. ensure patient-relevance).	▪ Insights on different design options – e.g. recall periods, item format, response scoring	Integrate patient preferences regarding elements of the PRO measure e.g. – instructions, layout, and font-size
Step 5. Refine the PRO measure's content: cognitive debriefing/content validation panels	▪ Confirm that focus and emphasis of the PRO measure are appropriate – language clarity, scoring, formatting.	▪ Feedback on psychometric validation study designs/protocol ▪ Confirm content validity of the prototype PRO measure (i.e. content comprehensiveness, and comprehensibility).	Incorporate patient preferences regarding the content elements – instructions, layout, font-size, number of items. Integrate mixed or quantitative approaches e.g. IRT analyses, descriptive analysis
Step 6. Explore the PRO measure's practicality and applicability	▪ Define relevant aspects of practicality/applicability to consider in pilot testing.	▪ Insights on feasibility of PRO measure for use in different settings (e.g. routine clinic).	Use final cognitive debrief interview round for pilot for efficiency. Perform descriptive analysis of responses
Step 7. Fine-tune the PRO measure, evaluate item performance, establish scoring algorithms	▪ Support interpretation of psychometric results. ▪ Item revision or deletion decision-making ▪ Reconcile frictions between different types of evidence e.g. qualitative vs. mathematical modelling.	▪ Confirm selection of final items in PROMs; proposed scoring algorithms.	Apply IRT analysis on the PRO measure e.g. evaluate scaling, and development of scoring algorithms
Step 8. Generate psychometric evidence and other supportive information	▪ Support development of clinical significance criteria ▪ Provide patient perspective on the totality of psychometric evidence ▪ Support patient-friendly dissemination of research findings – manuscripts / conference presentations.	▪ Feedback on adequacy of psychometric evidence vis-à-vis intended use of PRO measure	Continue life-cycle management of PRO measure – regularly review content validity, assess invariance in new settings of use.

Fig. 2.1 Roadmap for PRO measure development

As a minimum, the development of a new PRO measure needs to include the following steps:

Step 1. Define objectives of development of the PRO measure.
Step 2. Generate hypothesis and conceptualise the PRO measure: disease model/hypothetical conceptual physico-phsychosocial model.
Step 3. Gather and select item concepts: concept elicitation/qualitative research.
Step 4. Design and build the PRO measure: content definition/item generation.
Step 5. Refine the PRO measure's content: cognitive debriefing/content validation panels.
Step 6. Explore the PRO measure's practicality and applicability.
Step 7. Fine-tune the PRO measure, evaluate item performance, establish scoring algorithms.
Step 8. Generate psychometric evidence and other supportive information.

Step 1: Define Objectives of Development of the PROM

Clear objectives need to be articulated at the start of a PRO measure development programme addressing the context of use, i.e. routine clinical practice or clinical research, and the target population, i.e. condition/level of disease severity. This may be indeed influenced by a higher-level imperative such as a target product profile (TPP) of a drug, or an outcomes framework, in clinical practice.

Step 2: Generate Hypothesis and Conceptualise the PROM: Disease Model/Hypothetical Conceptual Physico-Psychosocial Model

Review of Literature and PROMs

The development of a new PRO measure requires a clear rationale which contributes to the definition and measurement of the construct under assessment. Strong theoretical basis for an instrument is essential in subsequent measure development steps, e.g. the assessment of construct validity (Bond 2004). A comprehensive review of the literature on the disease condition, its impacts and existing PRO measures is a good starting point. This may facilitate understanding of the need for assessing PROs as well as identify inadequacies in the existing measures in the context of the target population. Specifically, a literature review at this point may focus on the following topics:

Disease Burden

An understanding of the disease and its burden should, as a minimum, cover:

- The natural history of the disease.
- Major clinical features associated with a disease including comorbidities.
- Characteristics of the patient population in terms of demographic and clinical characteristics.

- Treatment guidelines as well as available current treatment options; identify the symptoms associated with the condition and their progression over time.
- The impacts of the disease on patient health status and quality of life and its progression over time.

The results of the literature review can be presented in a disease model which should provide an overview of the current knowledge about the disease.

Appraisal of Relevant PROMs

The PRO measures are evaluated in the context of a specific patient population focusing to understand:

- Existing PRO measures that have been used in in the target patient population.
- How well existing PRO measures address the concepts of interest in the specific patient population
- Psychometric evidence available for each PRO supporting validity in target population.
- Evidence gaps in psychometric information given intended use of PRO measure (i.e. for measures intended for use in regulatory settings, FDA standards on PRO measures can be used for comparison).

Results of appraisal may be presented in tabular form. Researchers have developed their own approaches to scoring each instrument in order to make the gap analysis process more structured (Valderas et al. 2008).

Development of Hypothetical Conceptual Framework

The next step is to draft a hypothetical conceptual framework for the measures, building on a thorough understanding of the PRO concepts of interest and related measures, from the insights and knowledge gathered from the previous steps, and taking into account the measurement objectives. It is critical that the development of the conceptual framework precedes the actual drafting and development of the instrument. See Fig. 3.1 for an example of a conceptual framework.

Step 3: Gather and Select Item Concepts: Concept Elicitation/ Qualitative Research

At the beginning of Step 3, it is assumed that the existing evidence on the PRO concepts of interest and related measures, as well as gaps, are well characterised and understood. Given the objectives of the PRO measurement, the process of defining and gathering content for the instrument can begin. Key activities in this stage include reflecting on the hypothesised conceptual framework with reference to what is to be measured, undertaking qualitative research to understand the patient's perspective (i.e. experiences, understanding and descriptions) and generating/developing the prototype instrument.

Eliciting Patient Input: Investigating the Experience of Patients Using Qualitative Research Methods

Patient input and involvement at this stage of the PRO measure development are critical, particularly in the identification of relevant item concepts and their wording/formulation. This is typically done using qualitative research methods, a research framework appropriate for gaining insights into beliefs, views and conceptual understanding held by subjects on an issue (Pope and Mays 2008). For instance, in the context of PRO measure development work, semi-structured interviews or focus groups may be carried out in the target patient population to explore and understand the various symptoms and impacts experienced by patients and the way these are described by the patients.

Various aspects are key to the validity, representativeness and usefulness of qualitative research findings for PRO measure development, including (1) inclusion of a diverse study population in terms of key clinical and demographic characteristics, e.g. severity of the condition, gender and age, in line with the PROM's target population, and (2) evidence of concept saturation, i.e. that all aspects of the concepts of interest important to the patients were captured (Food and Drug Administration 2009; Kerr et al. 2010). Please see Box 2.1 for further considerations in qualitative research in the context of PRO work.

Box 2.1 Undertaking Rigorous Qualitative Research to Understand Patients' Perspective

1. *Triangulate multiple data collection methods*

Triangulating multiple qualitative research methods such as focus groups and interviews is important in ensuring the validity and rigour of findings in qualitative research (Whittemore et al. 2001). In this way, the data collected is enriched by the strengths of each method. For instance, while interviews enable in-depth insights and greater disclosure, focus groups offer unique data through the interaction among subjects (Brod et al. 2009). Alternatively, surveys with open-ended questions may be used to confirm findings from a larger number of participants at a relatively lower cost.

2. *Data collection procedures should follow a structured process*

To facilitate data collection, a topic guide may need to be developed. This serves as an important aide to the researcher in guiding interviews or focus groups, especially probing on issues omitted by the patient which are known to be important from previous studies. During interviews, patients may be encouraged to elaborate more on their answers by probing them for reasons why or asking them for specific examples in their narratives. As a practical approach, the results from the focus groups/interviews may be used to inform questions in an open survey.

(continued)

Box 2.1 (continued)

Besides traditional approaches—face-to-face interviews and focus groups—other alternatives may be explored:

- Bespoke stand-alone online discussion boards may be developed. Discussion boards are typically used as platforms for Internet forums, allowing text-based discussions among any number of members and guests, and are managed by an administrator. In order to include only patients recruited to the study in discussions, participants will be given a username and password, for accessing the discussion board.
- One-on-one or group chats using online instant messaging platforms such as Skype, Windows Live Messenger, WhatsApp, WeChat, Viber and FaceTime.

3. *Analysis of data should be transparent and should ensure credibility*

A structured process is required in the analysis of qualitative data as part of PRO measure development. Good documentation is critical given that in some cases such evidence may be requested by regulatory agencies—where such PROs are being used in registration trials.

Thematic analysis is an approach most frequently used for data analysis during PRO measure development, due to its data-driven nature. Analyses commence without any preconceived theory; instead a framework is developed from the data as analysis proceeds, driving further data analysis and data collection (Braun and Clarke 2006). Issues emerging from the qualitative study analysis of the data transcripts are then organised as themes and subthemes. This could then be further developed into new items for a measure or could then support the selection of relevant item content from item banks.

Step 4: Design and Build the PROM: Content Definition/Item Generation

The major task in PROM design and building phase is to translate the conceptual framework and the content gathered from the qualitative research or other sources in the previous stages into a prototype measure. Transparency on the source and crafting of items is important for content validity, making it necessary to have a clear and structured process (Lynn 1986). Ideally, item crafting should be carried out by a multidisciplinary team comprised of experts in clinical research and patient outcome measurement. Criteria relating to the inclusion of content, wording of the actual items, and other elements of the PROM (i.e. layout, formatting, response options, instructions), should be clearly spelt out to guide the process. For example, issues with a prevalence of 5% or more during the qualitative research, or those regarded as relevant to certain subgroups based on age, gender or disease subtype, may be included (Streiner and Norman 2008). Key language considerations may include (1) drafting items based on language used by patients and avoiding technical jargons, (2) ensuring appropriate readability, (3) assessing a single concept only in each item and (4) ensuring response formats are appropriate for each item (DeVellis 2016; Patrick et al. 2011a).

Step 5: Refine the PROM's Content: Cognitive Debriefing/Content Validation Panels

The appropriateness of a newly crafted prototype PROM should be confirmed, based on assessment of how well the content (i.e. items, response options, instructions, etc.) is understood as well as the comprehensiveness of content in covering the underlying concept (Patrick et al. 2011a). This is best achieved using cognitive interviews although, for contexts other than medicines development programmes, content validation expert panels are equally appropriate.

Cognitive Interviews

Unlike in the qualitative research in previous phases which was exploratory, cognitive interviews are highly structured and are confirmatory. The focus is on four stages of cognitive processing in relation to the information in the PROM, including (1) comprehension or understanding of instructions, items and response options, (2) how memories relevant to the items are recollected, (3) evaluation of retrieved information and supplementing this where necessary and (4) selection response from options provided (Tourangeau 1984).

The Cognitive Interviews (CIs) are performed using two main techniques, 'think aloud' and 'verbal probing' techniques. In 'think aloud' technique, subjects are asked to verbalise interpretation of each item and their thinking process as they complete the questionnaire (Brod et al. 2009). In verbal probing, the interviewer uses additional probes, to identify issues in the PROM including relevance, length of questionnaire or potential gaps in the content (Patrick et al. 2011a).

Cognitive interviews are done iteratively, whereby, following a wave of two to three interviews, the PROM is revised to rectify issues identified; this is then followed by further CIs. Lack of any new problems identified as a result of further CIs is an indication of complete relevance.

The results from CI can be presented in form of summary tables including an overview on issues and problems identified in relation to cognitive processing aspects (as outlined above). In addition, an item matrix should be used to capture all revisions made as well as justification for such changes (Food and Drug Administration 2009).

Expert Panel for Content Validation

Expert panels comprised of clinicians, patients and PRO experts/psychometricians may be used to establish the appropriateness and relevance of a PROM's content. Expert panels of 5–7 members are asked to examine various elements in a PROM, including relevance, language clarity, comprehensiveness and response options.

The expert panels should be given adequate guidance on the exercise. For instance, a questionnaire can be used to collect information on the ratings for each element, prior to panel discussions. Panel discussions can then be conducted covering all elements of a PROM until consensus is reached among experts.

Results from the expert panels can be summarised using inter-rater agreement statistics (e.g. Kappa Coefficient, Intra-class correlation coefficient) and content validity index, for the item ratings while the qualitative feedback and other aspects discussed can be captured and presented via a summary table.

Step 6: Explore PROM's Practicality and Applicability

Aspects related to a PROMs practicality such as the aesthetics and design, ease of completion and time required for completion, as well as usefulness in addressing issues relevant to patients, have implications for the respondent burden associated with a PROM (Thornicroft and Slade 2000). The effort required to administer a measure as well as processing of the collected data is an equally important aspect of a measure's practicality. Broadly, practicality is of greater concern in routine clinical practice, where there might be particular constraints on time and monetary resources (Higginson and Carr 2001).

A pilot study should be carried out to explore such issues; typically, this is implemented through a small cross-section study design (~e.g. including 15 patients), where study participants complete the new instrument and a supplementary questionnaire assessing item comprehension and relevance, ease of completion and time to completion of the new measure. Possible additions to the measure may also be explored. Furthermore, problems encountered in completing the new instrument reflected in missing item responses or errors in completion can be noted. Items highlighted as unclear or causing any difficulties may be reviewed.

Step 7: Fine-Tune the PROM, Evaluate Item Performance and Establish Scoring Algorithms

Once the qualitative development of a PRO measure is finalised, the next critical task is to establish internal validity and determine how scale scores will be generated. This requires establishing a measurement model, identifying and eliminating poorly performing items and developing a scoring algorithm.

A measurement model operationalises the relationship between the underlying concept(s) and the items in a PRO measure, as defined in the conceptual framework (Lohr 2002), thus linking the scores to the underlying concept(s) (Byrne 2011). Various statistical techniques that differ in terms of their assumptions about the target concept are used in exploring measurement models, including item-total correlation analysis, multivariate regression analysis, scale score distribution statistics (i.e. mean, median, skewness, ceiling/floor effects), exploratory factor analysis (EFA), confirmatory factor analysis (CFA) and item response theory modelling. EFA is by far the most widely used, while CFA and IRT are relatively new, offering new capabilities (see Appendix for further details on EFA, and Box 2.2 for further details on CFA and IRT). Item response theory (IRT) modelling should be considered for all PRO measures, where appropriate, irrespective of other statistical modelling techniques used. Among other strengths of IRT analyses, insights in terms of hierarchical ordering of the items vis-à-vis the underlying concept are most helpful for achieving high precision and optimal measure targeting (Prieto et al. 2003; Bond and Fox 2015).

Alongside the analyses described above, it is standard practice to simultaneously evaluate how well the individual items function in contributing to measurement of the underlying concepts. Items not adding to the measurement should be considered for removal albeit with much care. A systematic and transparent process as well as clear criteria needs to be in place to support item deletion. Such decisions should not solely rely upon results of mathematical modelling but should also weigh on the qualitative evidence (Coste et al. 1997). For example, importance of a theme/issue to patients, overlaps with other items, conceptual scope of scale, relevance of an item to overall definition of concept (Guyatt et al. 1993). As a minimum, any item deletion should not negatively harm content validity.

The analyses specified in this phase can be implemented based on data from cross-sectional designs, or based on a single assessment or pooled data from longitudinal and other study designs.

This step of the roadmap, in particular, offers great opportunities for employing mixed methods approaches, enhancing the content validity, improving acceptability and the appropriateness of PRO measures. For example, clinicians or patients could be involved in defining concepts and appropriate domains, as well as item evaluation, using methods such as Delphi technique and group concept mapping.

Further, the procedures to be followed in calculating scores for scale and subscales should be provided, based on sound evidence as well as other considerations. Evidence supporting measurement model including results of CFA, IRT and item-level analyses is useful for establishing scoring algorithms. For example, a recommendation to have domain as well as overall scores must be underpinned by data supporting unidimensionality (i.e. that all items relate to a single concept) as well as potential grouping of items, which may come from a bi-factor model analysis.

A consideration in scoring is whether the contribution of each item to the scale or subscale scores is equal or differs. Although most widely used multi-item PRO measures assume equal weighing of items, there may be instances where assigning different weights to items is appropriate or even attractive to enhance predictive accuracy. However, the gains in terms of better predictive accuracy from such weighting should be balanced against its added complexity and administrative burden.

Various transformations may be applied on the raw scores, to facilitate score interpretation and comparison with other PRO measures. For example, raw scores can be standardised to generate z-scores or T-scores. A z-score expresses the raw score in standard deviation units and has a mean of zero and a standard deviation of 1 (Streiner and Norman 2008). Further transformation or centring of the z-score to a mean of 50 and a SD of 10 generates T-scores. For example, the PROMIS item banks use a T-score metric, normed (or anchored) on the US general population, which has a mean score of 50 and SD of 10 (Liu et al. 2010).

Box 2.2 Advanced Techniques Used in Fine-Tuning PRO Measures

Techniques with foundations in structural equation modelling (SEQM) and item response theory (IRT) offering greater insights on the underlying concept (latent variable) are now available and are increasingly being applied in PROM development. This has allowed re-conceptualisation of traditional attributes (assessed under classical test theory), as well as definition of properties not typically or readily evaluated under CTT.

Structural Equation Modelling

SEQM takes a confirmatory approach in evaluating statistical models involving causal interrelationships among variables, while explicitly capturing measurement error in the both explanatory and dependent variables (Byrne 2011). The framework accommodates both observable (or indicator) and unobservable (latent) variables.

SEQM-based methods are extremely flexible and may have various advantages, including (1) flexibility on how variables and their errors interrelate, (2) availability of statistical criteria for evaluating fit of data to a specified structure and (3) possibility to make direct comparisons among alternative structures (DeVellis 2016). A common application of SEQM methods is in testing hypothesised measurement models for PROMs, i.e. the extent to which observed variables (items in PROM) are linked to their underlying target concept, in CFA models.

In addition to pure hypothesis testing purposes, as in CFA, SEQM-based factor analyses may also support exploratory analyses, whereby the factor structure or the data (i.e. the PROM) can be iteratively changed, until fit is achieved. Inferences in SEQM-based factor analyses are based on goodness of fit, the significance of the individual item parameters (loadings) and magnitude of the residuals (i.e. residuals of 0.05 are indicative of good fit) (Byrne 2011). See Appendix—Technical Notes 2 "Suggestions for Statistical Analysis in PRO Development Work".

Item Response Theory

The item response theory offers a framework for scaling unidimensional instruments. The model expresses the probability of choosing a particular response to an item as a function of the relative difference between the severity level assessed by an item and that of the respondent, respectively. As both are measured on a common linear scale, this represents the distance between the item location and respondents location on the single linear scale of the latent variable (Tennant and Conaghan 2007). The relationship between the latent variable and the item responses follows a monotonic logistic ogive function, reflected in the item characteristic curve (ICC) (Wright and Masters 1982). This is similar to the curve representing a typical binary logistic function.

Box 2.2 (continued)

The Rasch model is based on core assumptions of unidimensionality and local independence, such that once the single latent variable (ϑ) is accounted for, no further relationship should exist between any two items (Reeve and Mâsse 2004). This gives rise to a probabilistic Guttman pattern whereby, for any given item, persons with greater severity (ability) should have a higher probability of choosing a higher category on an item in comparison to persons with less severity; the opposite also applies that for a given person, the probability of choosing a 'higher category' should be higher for items at lower severity level than those at a higher severity level for any person (Tennant et al. 2004). The steps involved in performing this analysis are described in Appendix—Technical Notes 4 "Performing Rasch Analysis".

Step 8: Generate Psychometric Evidence and Other Supportive Information

The validity of a PRO measure encompasses the evaluative judgement of the degree to which empirical evidence and theoretical rationales support the trustworthiness of interpretations and actions based on scale scores (Messick 1988). Such score inferences are specific to a particular context of use. Although a distinction is often made between content validity, criterion validity and construct validity, responsiveness and other attributes, these are strongly interdependent. The various properties generally reflect different forms of evidence supportive of the credibility, accuracy and dependability of a measure, as aspects of a holistic concept of construct validity (Streiner and Norman 2008).

Thus, the final step in the roadmap is dedicated to gathering different types of evidence to demonstrate measurement capabilities, including supporting score interpretations, of a PRO measure, including construct validity, reliability (i.e. precision), responsiveness (i.e. longitudinal validity), and clinical significance criteria.

Validity

The current section focuses on construct validity; key considerations for content validity are addressed in steps 1–5 of the roadmap, while criterion validity is considered to have limited relevance for PROMs.

Clear hypothesis relating to the expected outcome on the scores in different situations or how the scores may correlate with other variables needs to be tested to assess validity.

For example, hypothesis may include (1) testing whether 'patients with more severe disease would be expected to show greater HRQoL impairment', which would provide evidence discriminatory abilities of the PROM, or (2) testing whether 'the PROM scores correlate with scores from similar PROMs and do not correlate with dissimilar concept', as evidence for convergence and divergence validity.

Importantly, the patient population in which validity evidence is generated should be heterogeneous (in terms of the levels of the target concept) and should be similar to the target population for the PROM in terms of clinical and demographic characteristics such as age, gender and key disease characteristics. Preferably validity evidence should be generated based on the same mode of administration and setting as the intended use of the PROM, although there is cumulative evidence suggesting that mode of administration has a limited impact on measurement properties (Muehlhausen et al. 2015).

Reliability

Internal consistency and test-retest reliability are the most relevant forms of reliability for PROMs. In observer-rated measures, other forms of reliability such as inter-rater may also be relevant. Data from cross-sectional or longitudinal (i.e. single assessment or pooled data) designs are adequate for assessing internal consistency. Cronbach's alpha which represents the proportion of a scale's total variance that is attributable to a common source, i.e. the target concept (DeVellis 2016), is the most widely used test of internal consistency. Other tests such as item-total correlations are also useful.

Assessment of test-retest requires a longitudinal study design, where participants complete the new instrument on at least two assessments. The duration of follow-up between baseline and follow-up needs to be long enough to prevent practice effect but as short as possible so that the condition should have remained stable (Salek and Luscombe 1992). An anchor variable may help to ensure that the patient's condition has not changed. Test-retest reliability is determined by measuring the level of agreement in the baseline and follow-up scores assuming the patient's condition should have remained the same, using intra-class correlation coefficient (ICC) or other measures of absolute agreement. Reliability is interpreted as adequate if it ranges from 0.7 to 0.95 (Both et al. 2007).

Consideration of factors that may influence reliability should be made when interpreting reliability findings. As total variance is the denominator in the reliability equation, assuming measurement error is held constant, it may be possible to increase reliability of a measure simply by increasing total variability. This may occur as a result of increasing the number of items, sample heterogeneity and the number of response options, i.e. a phenomena referred to as *Spearman-Brown's prophecy* (Nunnally and Bernstein 1994).

Responsiveness

Responsiveness is assessed based on testing hypothesis relating to how PROM scores change in relation to changes in similar measures (Food and Drug Administration 2009). Such hypotheses may, for example, be related to differences in scores across patient groups according to an anchor variable such as a clinical measure of severity. In addition, hypotheses may also be based on expected score changes following treatment with interventions of known effectiveness.

The appropriateness of the follow-up duration should be based on disease area and PRO concept; otherwise this should be long enough to allow change in the patient's condition to have taken place. A longer follow-up duration may be expected for slow progressing conditions such as MS. The anchor variables used in assessing the status of the patient should show moderate correlation with the target PROM. Responsiveness is demonstrated in longitudinal study designs, e.g. data from clinical trials may be used to evaluate the responsiveness of PROMs.

Interpretability

Different forms of evidence including score categorisation (or banding system) or minimal clinically important differences (MCID) are useful in interpretation of PROMs. Score categorisations establish ranges of PROM scores corresponding to different levels of the condition, i.e. mild, moderate or severe levels (Prinsen et al. 2010). MCID, on the other hand, reflects the smallest change considered important to patients (Revicki et al. 2008).

Score interpretation information may be generated based on different approaches including (1) score sample distribution characteristics, (2) referencing to an external anchor and (3) qualitative research, e.g. patient interviews or expert panels.

- Distribution-based approaches apply measures of dispersion and other score distribution characteristics to define interpretation criteria. MICD is given as half-standard deviation of the scores or standard error of measurement (Norman et al. 2003).
- Anchor approaches use an external variable to assess change taking place in the patient's health status and to group patients according to this; then score distribution statistics such as mean and 95% CI are used to define score interpretation criteria. As a prerequisite, the variable used as an anchor must show good correlation with the target PROM. For example, mean change scores in the group defined as having smallest change in their condition provide an estimate of MCID (Wyrwich et al. 2005).
- Qualitative research approaches such as interviews in the target patient population may be used to prospectively define interpretation criteria on scores, e.g. score changes patients consider meaningful.

Data to support exploration/testing of criteria for absolute scores can be obtained from cross-sectional designs or alternatively single time-point assessment or pooled data from longitudinal designs. Similar designs are appropriate for distribution-based change score criteria (MCID) calculation. In contrast, anchor-based MCID requires longitudinal designs.

For anchor-based approaches, MCID analyses are similar to responsiveness testing—different metrics based on the magnitude of change in scores relating to different patient groups according to anchor variables are assessed. A triangulating of multiple anchors is recommended in establishing MCID (Guyatt et al. 2002).

Cross-Cutting Emergent Approaches

Patient Engagement

The participation of patients in PRO measure development research is widely acknowledged as being critical to the process and outcomes of research, in terms of acceptability, relevance, validity and patient centricity (de Wit et al. 2015). Patient-centricity objectives require that such participation goes beyond the traditional role of patients as research subjects, into an emergent role of partner/collaborator in order to actively incorporate the patient perspective into the research process (Frank et al. 2015). Specifically, this emergent approach to participation—also referred to as 'patient engagement'—may serve to inform decisions about research questions, study design and practical aspects of research implementation (Frank et al. 2015).

In practice, the nature of such engagement and the phase of PRO measure development are variable. de Wit et al. (2015) described different levels of patient participation in research, such as *information, consultation, advice, collaboration* and *control* (Frank et al. 2015). At the lowest level, 'information' communication is one way, and there is hardly any patient input into the research process. At the 'consultation' or 'advice' levels, some form of patient input is included, informing specific aspects, at particular phase(s) of research, e.g. ranking and prioritising HRQL issues/domains identified through interviews during content development. A patient advisory board may be assembled to provide guidance and input at critical points during the research. At higher levels of participation, 'collaboration' and 'control', there is a deliberate effort to retain a patient perspective in the research, for example, through inclusion of a patient research partner (PRP) on the research team. At the highest level 'control', the PRPs have equal say on the direction of the research as researchers.

Successful patient engagement requires various foundational elements (de Wit et al. 2015): (1) adequate preparation and planning which should include training of the PRP in PROs, and provision of appropriate information; (2) establishment of clearly defined 'communication channels' between patients and researcher partners such as face to face meetings, emails or online sharing; (3) the necessary resources and support, infrastructure and finances to facilitate patient engagement; and (4) commitment by the research team to ensuring that meaningful patient participation takes place.

Patient/public engagement in the research process has emerged as a formal requirement for many programmes and funding agencies, including the Patient-Centered Outcomes Research Institute (PCORI) in the USA, the Canadian Institutes of Health Research (CIHR) in Canada and the National Institute for Health Research (NIHR) in the UK, as well as the EU Innovative Medicines Initiative (Haywood et al. 2015).

In general, Patient engagement (PE) offers an opportunity to improve the science of PRO measure development and to reinforce the patient centredness of the process (Haywood et al. 2015; Forsythe et al. 2014). For example, PE may facilitate identification of topics/areas for future research, development of optimal study design, selection of appropriate outcomes/domains to include in a PRO instrument and clarification of patients' description of symptoms. PE may serve various functions at different stages of PRO development, such as (1) setting the research agenda and developing study hypotheses, during planning and preparatory stages; (2) providing feedback on draft study materials, including wording/phrasing of questions/topic guides; (3) feedback on conducting pilot interviews/focus group discussions; (4) recruitment of patients; (5) interpretation of data collected, e.g. qualitative data from patients, statistical results; and (6) reconciliation of tensions between various types and pieces of information during PRO development work.

Use of Social Networking Sites

The current universal proliferation of social media such as Facebook, YouTube, Twitter and blogs as an integral aspect of everyday communication has transformed the way patients and patient support groups organise and undertake their core activities, such as fundraising, addressing the psychological support needs of members or advancing their research agenda (Baldwin et al. 2011). Online patient social networks have now become more dynamic and have given rise to new forms of data (Baldwin et al. 2011; Frost et al. 2011). For example, Facebook has over 620 breast cancer groups, with a total membership of over one million (Bender et al. 2011). Other platforms (http://www.dmetrics.com) have registered over 2.5 billion health-related postings. A recent review (Hamm et al. 2013) cited up to 284 studies evaluating the impact of social media on patient and caregiver populations, suggesting a growing application of social media in health-related research. Social media has been utilised for various purposes, including (1) recruiting patients with rare diseases to investigate health status and behaviours related to treatment (Tweet et al. 2011; DiBenedetti et al. 2013), (2) public evaluation of symptoms and effectiveness of treatments (http://curetogether.com/blog/about/) and (3) as a rich source of insight into the views of patients on their disease experiences and on their treatments (Gustafson and Woodworth 2014).

A number of PRO measures have been developed or validated using social media (e.g. the Hyperhidrosis Quality of Life Index, the Insomnia Impact Questionnaire and the Multiple Sclerosis Rating Scale). However, these have not been used in medicine regulatory settings (Rothman et al. 2015; Kamudoni et al. 2015).

In PRO development work, social media may be employed in various ways (Rothman et al. 2015): first, supporting recruitment of patients, especially those who are otherwise hard to reach. Second, social media may offer a rich source of data, e.g. discussions on blogs and other social networking sites may be helpful in identification major disease symptoms, impacts and side effects of treatment. Further, as a tool for data collection, social media allows a two-way communication. There is a strong expectation that use of social media may offer potential savings in terms of time and resources associated with data collection, although this is yet to be demonstrated.

Assessing the suitability and appropriateness of different social media channels requires consideration of various aspects: (1) the purpose for using social media, e.g. patient recruitment/data collection, (2) anonymity requirements for the research and (3) how well patients in a channel represents the target population (Leidy and Murray 2013). The different social media channels have demonstrated heterogeneity in this regard. For example, in contrast to tweets and blogs, patient-powered research networks (PPRN) such as PatientsLikeMe tend to have more structured capture of information including demographic characteristics, medication and diagnoses as well as a outcomes (Leidy and Murray 2013). For instance, the level of motivation for research participation and chance for a correct diagnosis is also likely to be different between an approach targeting general Facebook and Google+ users according to their posts/'likes' and using PPRN or specific dedicated users.

There remain key obstacles to the use of social media in PRO development work. There is no precedence within medicines' regulatory processes for use of PRO measures developed and validated using social media channels. There is need for consensus on procedures and appropriate methods for obtaining informed consent that is relevant for social media. Respect for privacy and self-disclosure must be balanced against the need for verifying both the identity and diagnoses of the patients. The latter may, for example, be addressed by either asking patients to provide clinical information from their doctors or asking them for permission for researchers to contact their doctors directly. Finally, there is no clear best practice or research guidance on data confidentiality standards, for anonymous data sourced directly from social media such as blogs, tweets and forums. Also, no mechanism for verifying the quality and trustworthiness of such data—where the identity of the person supplying the data is not reported—is available (Rothman et al. 2015).

Appendix: Technical Notes

Practical Considerations in Study Design During PRO Development

Sample Size

Sample size considerations differ between qualitative and quantitative research. In the former, it is not possible to determine the needed sample size prior to data collection; rather sample adequacy is determined in the course of data collection. Data collection continues until 'saturation' has been reached, which reflects a situation where further data collection (e.g. interviews) is not yielding new data (Kerr et al. 2010). On the other hand, in quantitative research, sample size is dependent on the particular statistical analysis performed. Required sample size will reflect the intended power of analysis, the magnitude of effect size to be observed and the chosen level of significance and reliability of measurement (Lipsey 1990). Exploratory studies, where the magnitude of the effect size and reliability are unknown a priori, may present some challenges in this regard. A useful recommendation is to use a sample matrix based on key disease or treatment characteristics for a particular disease, where each subcategory (each cell) should have at least 15 subjects (Johnson et al. 2011). For initial estimates of reliability and validity, at least 200 subjects are recommended (Frost et al. 2007a). If a test-retest correlation of 0.85 is observed with a sample size of 100, the 95% confidence interval is 0.78–0.90, while a sample size of 150 would narrow this to 0.8–0.89 (Johnson et al. 2011).

Rules of thumb on sample size requirements for correlation analysis and factor analysis vary in their guidance, ranging from 5 to 20 observations per variable with more suggestion above and below this ratio (Costello and Osborne 2005). However, the minimum sample size required for accurate recovery of the population factor pattern matrix is influenced by many factors including the distribution and reliability of the variables, degree of association among variables, communalities and degree to which factors are overidentified (Reise et al. 2000; Schmitt 2011). Thus power and precision ought to be core considerations in parametric estimation-based factor methods (Schmitt 2011), while in non-parametric approaches when communalities are high, sample size of 100 may be adequate (Reise et al. 2000).

Assessment of adequacy of sample size for a given statistical test should be made along with other key considerations relating to the sample, for instance, ensuring that the target population is adequately represented along with all important disease characteristics. Otherwise, appropriate tools should be applied to indicate the uncertainty surrounding estimates, e.g. using confidence intervals in presenting results.

Missing Data

Situations where a question or an entire questionnaire has not been completed are common during data collection in QoL research. The reason behind the missing data has an influence on choice of tools for dealing with the consequent problems in data analysis, for example, whether an item is skipped by mistake or due to its irrelevance. There are three main classifications of patterns of missing data: missing completely at random (MCAR), missing at random (MAR) and missing not at random (MNAR) (Fayers and Machin 2007). MCAR arises where the probability of having a missing item (questionnaire) is independent of previous or unobserved current and future scores. MAR occurs where missingness is dependent on known covariates and scores of previous items, but not on the unobserved scores. The third case relates to where the unobserved HRQoL influences the missingness. The presence of MAR and MCAR is not worrisome, as their impact on accurate measurement of HRQoL is minimal (Leidy et al. 1999). MNAR causes the greatest concern as its presence may lead to an over- or underestimation of HRQoL, highlighting the need for transparent approaches in addressing its presence.

There are no clear guidelines on the number of missing items to warrant the exclusion of an entire respondent's questionnaire from analyses although Streiner and Norman (2008) have mentioned a ceiling of 5% of items. However, it's worth noting that where Rasch scoring is applied, a higher number of missing items may be tolerated without much bias in measurement (Fayers and Machin 2007). On the other hand, in some situations (e.g. during instrument development work), data imputation to replace the missing data offers a viable alternative. This is done in various ways including using the last observed value carried forward, by calculating a simple mean or using regression methods (Fairclough 2010). Other more sophisticated imputation approaches such as hot-deck and Markov chain are capable of preserving variability in the data.

Strategies for preventing problems of missing data from rising should be considered, e.g. inviting the patients to cross-check their questionnaires to make sure all items are completed (~assuming paper-and-pencil in-person administration). Here electronic PRO administration may have advantages.

Suggestions for Statistical Analysis in PROM Development

Data should initially be explored through descriptive analysis of each variable, calculating measures of central tendency (mean, median), variability (SD) and interquartile range for continuous variable. Frequency counts for ordinal and categorical variables. Further analyses will involve making inferences based on various hypotheses tests. In order to reject a null hypothesis, observed probability of a false positive, type I error, as reflected in *P*-value, needs to be less than the required level of significance (α) (Altman et al. 2013). Most studies will use a level of significance (α) of 5%. Where several hypotheses need to be simultaneously tested, Bonferroni adjustment should be applied to the level of significance, as (α/k), where k is the number of tests (Fayers and Machin 2007).

- Testing for differences between two means should use independent or paired *t*-test, depending on whether the two means are mutually exclusive or are related. The Mann-Whitney and Wilcoxon tests are the non-parametric alternatives, respectively, for situations where assumptions of the *t*-tests are not met. These latter tests are somewhat more conservative.
- Hypothesis tests involving differences among more than two groups should be carried out using the ANOVA test. Where the core assumptions of this test are not met, particularly, the assumption of homogenous variances across group, the Kruskal-Wallis test should be used alternatively.
- Testing of hypotheses relating to associations between means of variables should be carried out based on Pearson's correlations. Where the data is not continuous, Spearman's rank correlation should be used.
- Polychoric correlations can be estimated in order to assess multicollinearity among items. This type of correlation produces consistent and robust results in ordinal data. They are based on the assumption that the variable is linear and continuous but divided up in a series of categories (Holgado-Tello et al. 2010). Multicollinearity is identified when correlation coefficients are 0.8 or greater.
- Possible influences on the magnitude of observed inter-item correlations including range of score values, homogeneity of items, distribution of the data

(particularly departures from normality) and existence of outliers in the data (Fayers and Machin 2007) should be explored. Normality assumption implies the absolute value of skewness not exceeding 3, while the absolute value of Kurtosis must not be greater than 7 (Ozer et al. 2009; Byrne 2011). While the former impacts on means, covariance tends to be vulnerable to Kurtosis values (Byrne 2011).

Further statistical analyses carried out during construct validation can use various forms of regression methods, modelling latent variables including exploratory factor analysis, confirmatory factor analysis and the Rasch model.

Performing Exploratory Factor Analysis

The aim is to identify the smallest number of interpretable factors explaining the covariation among items (Muthen and Muthén 2010). This involves first generating the variance-covariance matrix, followed by the estimation of the factors which entails putting together those items sharing the highest covariation. Subsequently, the initial factor solution is rotated in order to achieve a simple structure that is more interpretable, as the initial solution is not unique (DeVellis 2016).

To perform an EFA on the instrument, first a polychoric correlation matrix should be generated. This more appropriately takes into account the ordinality of the data and remains robust when data are skewed, in comparison to the conventional Pearson's correlation coefficients (Byrne 2011). The initial factor estimation can be carried out using a robust diagonally least squares estimator (WLSMV) which yields robust test statistics, parameter estimates and standard errors when indicator variables are categorical and where normality assumptions are violated (Byrne 2011). Rotation can be performed using the Geomin routine (~available in Mplus software, equivalents might be known by other names in other software), which allows correlation among factors. This rotation is particularly suitable for psychosocial domains known to be highly related (Lackey et al. 2003). Where the factors are not related, Geomin still performs well yielding results comparable to orthogonal rotation routines. Choice of the appropriate number of factors to be extracted will be based on the parallel analysis and will be confirmed by statistical goodness of fit measures (Schmitt 2011). Kaiser's rule, based on size of eigenvalues; scree plot, which is a graph of number of factors against eigenvalues; and parallel analysis, comparing actual against ones randomly generated, should also be reported. The following criteria can be applied:

- Kaiser's rule: factors with eigenvalues greater than are included (Kaiser (1960) in (DeVellis 2016)).
- Scree plot: all factors to the left of the 'ankle' are extracted, where there is a change in the slope.
- Parallel analysis: the last factor to be retained must have an eigenvalue greater than the one that would be produced randomly (Williams et al. 2010).

An advantage of factor estimation using Likelihood methods is the possibility to generate goodness of fit indices to explore how well hypothesised models fit data. These can be classified into three groups:

- Chi-square-based indices compare a single factor model against a model with the chosen number of factors (*k*). For the 'chi-goodness of fit test', a non-significant chi-statistic represents good fit (Lackey et al. 2003).
- Practical fit indices evaluate the proportionate improvement in the model by comparing a hypothesised model against a less restricted baseline model (Byrne 2011). For comparative fit index and Tucker-Lewis Index, values of below 0.9 and 0.95 indicate acceptable and adequate fit, respectively (Schmitt 2011).
- Absolute fit indices are based on analysis of residuals after fitting the model to the data. For Root Mean Square Error of Approximation (RMSEA), a value below 0.05 shows good fit, 0.08–0.1 mediocre fit and above 0.1 poor fit (Brown 2014). For the Standardized Root Mean Square Residual (SRMR), values lower than 0.05 indicate 'adequate fit' although values below 0.8 are still acceptable. The Weighted Root Mean Square Residual uses a cut-off value of 0.95 for good fit.

Performing Rasch Analysis

Appropriate fit to the Rasch model ensures that an PRO measure is sufficiently unidimensional and that it complies with conjoint measurement principles, a precondition for converting the data from the instrument into interval scales (Bond 2004). The intention of Rasch analysis, therefore, is to evaluate whether data have sufficient fit to the model to warrant such claims.

Demonstrating conformity to the Rasch model may have several advantages for a PRO instrument. First, ordinal scores may be transformed into interval-level logit scores using the RM—a requisite property for the calculation of effect sizes and other statistics in clinical research that is usually taken for granted (Reise and Haviland 2005). Second, by conceptualising measurement error as an item-level property, high reliability can be attained even with a shorter questionnaire, making it possible to minimise patient burden without compromising precision (Reeve et al. 2007). In addition, much more complex comparisons such as 'anchoring' or 'equating' may be easily carried out between an instrument and other instruments.

When assessing conformity to the Rasch model, its assumptions and properties involve the following:

1. Assessing whether the response categories are functioning optimally. *Average latent measure* across observations in a response category and *category thresholds* should monotonically increase with the category; each response category should have a distinct peak on the *category probability curve* graph reflecting the space along the latent variable where it is most probable (Linacre 1999). Category characteristic curves define the most likely response category for a specific per-

son location value on the latent variable. The category threshold indicates a location on the latent variable where the probability of selecting adjacent categories is equivalent (Linacre 1999).

2. Testing item and person fit to the model. This uses residuals obtained after fitting data to the model, calculating a fit residual statistic and an item-trait interaction chi-statistic. The residual statistic for items is calculated as the squared summation of the standardised residuals of the responses of all persons to an item (Andrich et al. 2012b). Fit residuals exceeding $| \pm 2.5|$ indicate poor fit (Andrich et al. 2012a). As the Rasch model does not distinguish between items and persons, the residual fit statistics for persons is calculated and interpreted in a similar way as the statistic for items (Bond and Fox 2015).
3. The item-trait interaction test of fit assesses the discrepancy between actual and model scores of class intervals (which group patients according to ability), visually reflected by discrepancies between the ICC and empirical counterpart. An item chi-value is generated by adding all standardised differences for class intervals (Andrich et al. 2012a).
4. Testing of overall model fit. Mean fit residual value of 0 and standard deviation of 1 reflect overall model fit (Shea et al. 2009). The item-trait interaction statistics for all items are summed up into total item-trait interaction statistic. Optimal fit is reflected in a non-significant statistic (chi-squared statistic, P-value >0.05). Good fit to the Rasch model implies that the hierarchical ordering of the items remains invariant across the different levels of disease severity assessed by the construct.
5. How well the instrument can differentiate persons according to disease severity should be assessed. This is reflected in the Person Separation Index (PSI) which reflects the proportion of variance explained by the model out of the total person variability (Wright and Masters 1982; Bond and Fox 2015). A PSI of 0.8 reflects capability to reliably distinguish patients into at least two groups of severity, e.g. high and low severity.
6. Assessing targeting of items. The item-person map is visually examined for adequacy in spread of the items along the breadth of the latent variable, and ideally there should not be large gaps between items (Wright and Masters 1982); mean location of persons should be close to 0 to match the item mean location centred at 0 logits (Gorecki et al. 2011).
7. Assessing unidimensionality. First, a principal component analysis should be carried out on the residuals after fitting the Rasch model. Unidimensionality is supported if the first component accounts for no more than 30% of the variance in the data and has an eigenvalue of 3 or less (Linacre 1998). A more stringent assessment of unidimensionality has been suggested by Smith (2002). Items are grouped according to their loading on the first residual factor, comprised of high positive and high negative loading items, respectively. Pairs of person estimates generated from the two item sets are compared using a series of t-tests. If the proportion of significant tests (or the lower bound of its confidence interval) exceeds 5%, unidimensionality is ruled out (Tennant and Pallant 2006).

8. The assumption of local independence can be assessed by examining the correlation matrix of the item residuals. Residual correlation exceeding 0.2–0.3 reflects a violation of this assumption. The magnitude of the response dependence is calculated as the shift in the latent variable range representing a given response choice on the dependent item, induced by a particular response choice on the independent item (Andrich et al. 2012b).
9. Assessing for invariance across demographic factors. Differential item functioning (DIF) can be assessed for key demographic factors using a two-way ANOVA test. A significant main effect (demographic variable) at a 0.05 level of significance, with Bonferroni adjustment, indicates presence of uniform DIF. On the other hand, a significant interaction effect (demographic variable X class interval representing ability groups along the latent trait), after Bonferroni adjustment, indicates non-uniform DIF (Andrich et al. 2012a). Identification of DIF requires a pure set of items, upon which the scale is anchored (Teresi and Fleishman 2007).

   Any action on DIF requires an understanding of its magnitude and impact. Magnitude indicates the difference between item difficulty estimates based on all patients and comparable estimates specific for each demographic group (Linacre 2009). The impact of the DIF on estimation of person estimates is assessed by comparing person estimates generated from the DIF-free items against estimates based on all items including those with DIF (Pallant and Tennant 2007). Using a *t*-test, significant results, at 0.05 level of significance, indicate that DIF has an impact. The Item Characteristic Curve (ICC) of the two series may also be useful in assessing whether the pairs of person ability estimates agree. Impact of DIF can also be explored by assessing whether the test characteristic curves (TCCs) from different demographic groups are comparable, i.e. whether there is a relationship between the raw score and the underlying latent variable varies across the demographic groups. Identical TCCs indicate the absence of impact of DIF on the total score (Edelen et al. 2006). The criterion for magnitude of DIF is also relevant for differential scale functioning.

References

Altman D, Machin D, Bryant T, Gardner M (2013) Statistics with confidence: confidence intervals and statistical guidelines. John Wiley & Sons, Hoboken

Andrich D, Sheridan B, Luo G (2012a) Interpreting RUMM 2030 analysis: part i dichotomous data. RUMM Laboratory, Perth

Andrich D, Humphry SM, Marais I (2012b) Quantifying local, response dependence between two polytomous items using the Rasch Model. Appl Psychol Meas 36(4):309–324

Baldwin M, Spong A, Doward L, Gnanasakthy A (2011) Patient-reported outcomes, patient-reported information from randomized controlled trials to the social web and beyond. Patient 4:11–17

Bender JL, Jimenez-Marroquin MC, Jadad AR (2011) Seeking support on facebook: a content analysis of breast cancer groups. J Med Internet Res 13(1). https://doi.org/10.2196/jmir.1560

Bond T (2004) Validity and assessment: a Rasch measurement perspective. Metodol Ciencias Del Comportamiento 5:179–194

Bond T, Fox CM (2015) Applying the Rasch Model: fundamental measurement in the human sciences. Routledge, London

Both H, Essink-Bot M-L, Busschbach J, Nijsten T (2007) Critical review of generic and dermatology-specific health-related quality of life instruments. J Investig Dermatol 127(12):2726–2739

Braun V, Clarke V (2006) Using thematic analysis in psychology. Qual Res Psychol 3(2): 77–101

Brod M, Tesler LE, Christensen TL (2009) Qualitative research and content validity: developing best practices based on science and experience. Qual Life Res 18(9):1263

Brown TA (2014) Confirmatory factor analysis for applied research. Guilford Publications, New York

Byrne B (2011) Structural equation modeling with mplus: basic concepts, applications, and programming. Routledge, New York. http://books.google.de/books?id=u58MPwAACAAJ

Coons SJ, Gwaltney CJ, Hays RD, Lundy JJ, Sloan JA, Revicki DA, Lenderking WR, Cella D, Basch E (2009) Recommendations on evidence needed to support measurement equivalence between electronic and paper-based patient-reported outcome (PRO) measures: ISPOR ePRO Good Research Practices Task Force report. Value Health 12(4):419–429

Coste J, Guillemin F, Pouchot J, Fermanian J (1997) Methodological approaches to shortening composite measurement scales. J Clin Epidemiol 50(3):247–252

Costello AB, Osborne JW (2005) Best practices in exploratory factor analysis: four recommendations for getting the most from your analysis. Pract Assess Res Eval 10(7):1–9

Dalal AA, Nelson L, Gilligan T, McLeod L, Lewis S, DeMuro-Mercon C (2011) Evaluating patient-reported outcome measurement comparability between paper and alternate versions, using the lung function questionnaire as an example. Value Health 14(5):712–720

DeVellis RF (2016) Scale development: theory and applications. Applied social research methods. SAGE Publications, Thousand Oaks. https://books.google.de/books?id=48ACCwAAQBAJ

DiBenedetti DB, Coles TM, Sharma T (2013) Recruiting patients with a rare blood disorder and their caregivers through social media. Value Health 16(3):A51

Dillman DA (2007) Mail and internet surveys: the tailored design method. Wiley, Hoboken

Edelen MO, Thissen D, Teresi JA, Kleinman M, Ocepek-Welikson K (2006) Identification of differential item functioning using item response theory and the likelihood-based model comparison approach: application to the mini-mental state examination. Med Care 44(11):S134–S142

Epstein RS (2000) Responsiveness in quality-of-life assessment: nomenclature, determinants, and clinical applications. Med Care 38(9 Suppl):II91

Fairclough DL (2010) Design and analysis of quality of life studies in clinical trials. CRC Press, Boca Raton

Fayers PM, Machin D (2007) Quality of life: the assessment, analysis and interpretation of patient-reported outcomes, 2nd edn. John Wiley & Sons, West Sussex

Food and Drug Administration (2009) Guidance for industry: patient-reported outcome measures: use in medical product development to support labeling claims. Fed Regist 74(235):65132–65133

Forsythe LP, Szydlowski V, Murad MH, Ip S, Wang Z, Elraiyah TA, Fleurence R, Hickam DH (2014) A systematic review of approaches for engaging patients for research on rare diseases. J Gen Intern Med 29(3):788–800

Frank L, Forsythe L, Ellis L, Schrandt S, Sheridan S, Gerson J, Konopka K, Daugherty S (2015) Conceptual and practical foundations of patient engagement in research at the patient-centered outcomes research institute. Qual Life Res 24(5):1033–1041

Frost J, Okun S, Vaughan T, Heywood J, Wicks P (2011) Patient-reported outcomes as a source of evidence in off-label prescribing: analysis of data from PatientsLikeMe. J Med Internet Res 13(1):e6

Frost MH, Reeve BB, Liepa AM, Stauffer JW, Hays RD, Mayo/FDA Patient-Reported Outcomes Consensus Meeting Group (2007a) What is sufficient evidence for the reliability and validity of patient-reported outcome measures? Value Health 10:S94–S105

Frost MH, Bonomi AE, Cappelleri JC, Schünemann HJ, Moynihan TJ, Aaronson NK (2007b) Applying quality-of-life data formally and systematically into clinical practice. Mayo Clin Proc 82(10):1214–1228

Gorecki C, Lamping DL, Nixon J, Brown JM, Cano S (2011) Applying mixed methods to pretest the pressure ulcer quality of life (PU-QOL) instrument. Qual Life Res 21(3):441–451

Gustafson DL, Woodworth CF (2014) Methodological and ethical issues in research using social media: a metamethod of human papillomavirus vaccine studies. BMC Med Res Methodol 14(1):127

Guyatt G, Walter S, Norman G (1987) Measuring change over time: assessing the usefulness of evaluative instruments. J Chronic Dis 40(2):171–178

Guyatt GH, Osoba D, Wu AW, Wyrwich KW, Norman GR (2002) Methods to explain the clinical significance of health status measures. Mayo Clin Proc 77(4):371–383

Guyatt GH, Feeny DH, Patrick DL (1993) Measuring health-related quality of life. Ann Intern Med 118(8):622–629

Hamm MP, Chisholm A, Shulhan J, Milne A, Scott SD, Given LM, Hartling L (2013) Social media use among patients and caregivers: a scoping review. BMJ Open 3(5). https://doi.org/10.1136/bmjopen-2013-002819

Haynes SN, Richard D, Kubany ES (1995) Content validity in psychological assessment: a functional approach to concepts and methods. Psychol Assess 7(3):238

Hays RD, Hadorn D (1992) Responsiveness to change: an aspect of validity, not a separate dimension. Qual Life Res 1(1):73–75

Haywood K, Brett J, Salek S, Marlett N, Penman C, Shklarov S, Norris C, Santana MJ, Staniszewska S (2015) Patient and public engagement in health-related quality of life and patient-reported outcomes research: what is important and why should we care? Findings from the first ISOQOL patient engagement symposium. Qual Life Res 24(5):1069–1076

Higginson IJ, Carr AJ (2001) Measuring quality of life: using quality of life measures in the clinical setting. BMJ 322(7297):1297

Holgado-Tello FP, Chacón-Moscoso S, Barbero-García I, Vila-Abad E (2010) Polychoric versus Pearson correlations in exploratory and confirmatory factor analysis of ordinal variables. Qual Quant 44(1):153–166

Johnson, C, N Aaronson, JM Blazeby, A Bottomley, P Fayers, M Koller, D Kuliś, et al. 2011. "The European Organization for Research and Treatment of Cancer: guidelines for developing questionnaire modules, 4th edn. Qual Life Res 2

Kamudoni P, Mueller B, Salek MS (2015) The development and validation of a disease-specific quality of life measure in hyperhidrosis: the Hyperhidrosis Quality of Life Index (HidroQOL©). Qual Life Res 24(4):1017–1027

Kerr C, Nixon A, Wild D (2010) Assessing and demonstrating data saturation in qualitative inquiry supporting patient-reported outcomes research. Expert Rev Pharmacoecon Outcomes Res 10(3):269–281

Kline P (1994) An easy guide to factor analysis. Taylor & Francis Group, London. http://books.google.co.uk/books?id=6PHzhLD-bSoC

Lackey NR, Sullivan JJ, Pett MA (2003) Making sense of factor analysis: the use of factor analysis for instrument development in health care research. SAGE Publications Ltd, London. http://books.google.co.uk/books?id=5Jyaa2LQWbQC

Leidy NK, Murray LT (2013) Patient-reported outcome (PRO) measures for clinical trials of COPD: the EXACT and E-RS. COPD: J Chron Obstruct Pulmon Dis 10(3):393–398

Leidy NK, Revicki DA, Genesté B (1999) Recommendations for evaluating the validity of quality of life claims for labeling and promotion. Value Health 2(2):113–127

Liang MH (2000) Longitudinal construct validity: establishment of clinical meaning in patient evaluative instruments. Med Care 38(9):II

Linacre JM (1998) Detecting multidimensionality: which residual data-type works best? J Outcome Meas 2:266–283

Linacre MH (1999) Investigating rating scale category utility. J Outcome Meas 3(2):103

Linacre JM (2009) A user's guide to WINSTEPS/MINISTEPS. Rasch-Model Computer Programs, Chicago. Winsteps.com

Lipsey MW (1990) Design sensitivity: statistical power for experimental research, 19th edn. SAGE Publication Ltd., London

Liu H, Cella D, Gershon R, Shen J, Morales LS, Riley W et al (2010) Representativeness of the patient-reported outcomes measurement information system internet panel. J Clin Epidemiol 63(11):1169–1178

Lohr KN (2002) Assessing health status and quality-of-life instruments: attributes and review criteria. Qual Life Res 11(3):193–205. https://doi.org/10.1023/a:1015291021312

Lynn MR (1986) Determination and quantification of content validity. Nurs Res 35(6):382–385

Messick S (1988) The once and future issues of validity: assessing the meaning and consequences of measurement. Test Valid 33:45

Muehlhausen W, Doll H, Quadri N, Fordham B, O'Donohoe P, Dogar N, Wild DJ (2015) Equivalence of electronic and paper administration of patient-reported outcome measures: a systematic review and meta-analysis of studies conducted between 2007 and 2013. Health Qual Life Outcomes 13(1):167

Muthen LK, Muthén BO (2010) Mplus user's guide, v. 6.1. Muthen and Muthen, UCLA, Los Angeles

Norman GR, Sloan JA, Wyrwich KW (2003) Interpretation of changes in health-related quality of life: the remarkable universality of half a standard deviation. Med Care 41(5):582

Norquist JM, Girman C, Fehnel S, DeMuro-Mercon C, Santanello N (2011) Choice of recall period for patient-reported outcome (PRO) measures: criteria for consideration. Qual Life Res 21:1013–1021

Nunnally JC, Bernstein IH (1994) Psychometric theory. McGraw-Hill, London. http://books.google.de/books?id=r0fuAAAAMAAJ

Ozer ZC, Firat MZ, Bektas HA (2009) Confirmatory and exploratory factor analysis of the caregiver quality of life index-cancer with Turkish samples. Qual Life Res 18(7):913–921

Pallant JF, Tennant A (2007) An introduction to the rasch measurement model: an example using the Hospital Anxiety and Depression Scale (HADS). Br J Clin Psychol 46(1):1–18

Patrick DL, Burke LB, Gwaltney CJ, Leidy NK, Martin ML, Molsen E, Ring L (2011a) Content validity – establishing and reporting the evidence in newly developed patient-reported outcomes (PRO) instruments for medical product evaluation: ISPOR PRO good research practices task force report: part 2 – assessing respondent understanding. Value Health 14(8):978–988

Patrick DL, Burke LB, Gwaltney CJ, Leidy NK, Martin ML, Molsen E, Ring L (2011b) Content validity – establishing and reporting the evidence in newly developed patient-reported outcomes (PRO) instruments for medical product evaluation: ISPOR PRO good research practices task force report: part 1 – eliciting concepts for a new PRO instrument. Value Health 14(8):967–977. https://doi.org/10.1016/j.jval.2011.06.014

Patrick DL, Deyo RA (1989) Generic and disease-specific measures in assessing health status and quality of life. Med Care 27:217–232

Pope C, Mays N (2008) Qualitative research in health care, 3rd edn. Wiley-Blackwell, Oxford. http://books.google.de/books?id=DMxS6R3s2a4C

Prieto L, Alonso J, Lamarca R (2003) Classical test theory versus Rasch analysis for quality of life questionnaire reduction. Health Qual Life Outcomes 1(1):27

Prinsen CAC, Lindeboom R, Sprangers MAG, Legierse CM, de Korte J (2010) Health-related quality of life assessment in dermatology: interpretation of Skindex-29 scores using patient-based anchors. J Invest Dermatol 130(5):1318–1322

Reeve BB, Hays RD, Chang CH, Perfetto EM (2007) Applying item response theory to enhance health outcomes assessment. Qual Life Res 16:1–3

Reeve BB, Mâsse LC (2004) Methods for testing and evaluating survey questionnaires. In: Presser S, Rothgeb JM, Couper MP, Lessler JT, Martin E, Martin J, Singer E (eds) Item response theory modeling for questionnaire evaluation. John Wiley & Sons, Inc, Hoboken, pp 247–273. https://doi.org/10.1002/0471654728.ch13

Reise SP, Haviland MG (2005) Item response theory and the measurement of clinical change. J Pers Assess 84(3):228–238

Reise SP, Waller NG, Comrey AL (2000) Factor analysis and scale revision. Psychol Assess 12(3):287

Revicki D, Hays RD, Cella D, Sloan J (2008) Recommended methods for determining responsiveness and minimally important differences for patient-reported outcomes. J Clin Epidemiol 61(2):102–109

Rothman M, Gnanaskathy A, Wicks P, Papadopoulos EJ (2015) Can we use social media to support content validity of patient-reported outcome instruments in medical product development? Value Health 18(1):1–4

Rothman ML, Beltran P, Cappelleri JC, Lipscomb J, Teschendorf B, F. D. A. Patient-Reported Outcomes Consensus Meeting Group the Mayo (2007) Patient-reported outcomes: conceptual issues. Value Health 10:S66–S75. https://doi.org/10.1111/j.1524-4733.2007.00269.x

Salek MS, Luscombe DK (1992) Health-related quality of life assessment: a review. J Drug Dev 5:137–137

Salek S (1998) Compendium of quality of life instruments, vol 4. Euromed Communications, Haslemere. http://books.google.de/books?id=2_LaAAAAMAAJ

Schmitt TA (2011) Current methodological considerations in exploratory and confirmatory factor analysis. J Psychoeduc Assess 29(4):304–321

Shea T, Tennant A, Pallant J (2009) Rasch model analysis of the Depression, Anxiety and Stress Scales (DASS). BMC Psychiatry 9(1):21

Smith EV (2002) Detecting and evaluating the impact of multidimensionality using item fit statistics and principal component analysis of residuals. J Appl Meas 3(2):205–231

Streiner DL, Norman GR (2008) Health measurement scales: a practical guide to their development and use. Oxford University Press, Oxford. http://books.google.co.uk/books?id=UbKijeRqndwC

Tennant A, Conaghan PG (2007) The Rasch Measurement Model in rheumatology: what is it and why use it? When should it be applied, and what should one look for in a Rasch paper? Arthritis Care Res 57(8):1358–1362

Tennant A, McKenna SP, Hagell P (2004) Application of Rasch analysis in the development and application of quality of life instruments. Value Health 7(Suppl 1):S22–S26

Tennant A, Pallant JF (2006) Unidimensionality matters. Rasch Measur Trans 20(1):1048–1051

Teresi JA, Fleishman JA (2007) Differential item functioning and health assessment. Qual Life Res 16:33–42

Terwee CB, Bot SDM, De Boer MR, van der Windt DAWM, Knol DL, Dekker J, Bouter LM, De Vet HCW (2007) Quality criteria were proposed for measurement properties of health status questionnaires. J Clin Epidemiol 60(1):34–42

Thornicroft G, Slade M (2000) Are routine outcome measures feasible in mental health? Qual Health Care 9(2):84–84

Tourangeau R (1984) Cognitive aspects of survey methodology: building a bridge between disciplines. In: Jabine TB et al (eds) Cognitive sciences and survey methods. Institute for Social and Economic Research, Essex, pp 73–100

Tweet MS, Gulati R, Aase LA, Hayes SN (2011) Spontaneous coronary artery dissection: a disease-specific, social networking community-initiated study. Mayo Clin Proc 86(9):845–850

Valderas JM, Ferrer M, Mendívil J, Garin O, Rajmil L, Herdman M, Alonso J (2008) Development of EMPRO: a tool for the standardized assessment of patient-reported outcome measures. Value Health 11(4):700–708

Ware JE, Kosinski M, Keller SD (1994) SF-36 physical and mental health summary scales: a user's manual. The Health Institute, Boston, MA

Whittemore R, Chase SK, Mandle CL (2001) Validity in qualitative research. Qual Health Res 11(4):522–537

Williams B, Onsman A, Brown T (2010) Exploratory factor analysis: a five-step guide for novices. J Emerg Primary Health Care 8(3):1–13 de Wit MPT, Kvien TK, Gossec L (2015) Patient participation as an integral part of patient-reported outcomes development ensures the representation of the patient voice: a case study from the field of rheumatology. RMD Open 1(1):e000129

Wright BD, Masters GN (1982) Rating scale analysis. Mesa Press, Chicago. http://books.google.de/books?id=ZfjFQgAACAAJ

Wynd CA, Schmidt B, Schaefer MA (2003) Two quantitative approaches for estimating content validity. West J Nurs Res 25(5):508–518

Wyrwich KW, Bullinger M, Aaronson N, Hays RD, Patrick DL, Symonds T (2005) Estimating clinically significant differences in quality of life outcomes. Qual Life Res 14(2):285–295

Part II

An Illustration of the New PRO Measure Development Roadmap Using Research in Hyperhidrosis as A Practical Example

3 Conceptualisation and Qualitative Development of a PRO Measure

The purpose of this and the subsequent three chapters is to provide a step-by-step guide of how the framework proposed in Chap. 2 could be implemented, using research carried out by our research group in hyperhidrosis, as an example. This chapter lays a foundation for the three practical chapters by providing some background information about hyperhidrosis, which is then summarised using a disease model diagram. Approaches used in the hypothesis generation process as well as concept elicitation qualitative research to gather and select item concepts that reflect the experience of patients in hyperhidrosis will be presented (Steps 2 to 3 in the roadmap). Methods used in the content definition/item generation process of the Hyperhidrosis Quality of Life Index (HidroQoL) will also be discussed in the current chapter (Step 4). Chapter 4 will discuss discuss how the appropriateness of a PRO's content is established and the subsequent steps to refine and eventually pretest the revised draft measure (Steps 5 and 6 of the roadmap).

Chapter 5 illustrates how a newly developed or existing measure could be fine-tuned using item response theory methods. This is followed by a case study on classical PRO measure validation to establish core psychometric properties, in chapter 6.

The rest of the chapter is organised under two sections. The first, Part I, presents a background and disease model for hyperhidrosis. The second, Part II, presents a case study, based on the qualitative development of the Hyperhidrosis Quality of Life Index, including hypothesis generation, item generation and selection, and the design and building of the measure.

Part I: Hyperhidrosis Disease—Disease Background

Primary hyperhidrosis is characterised by spontaneous excessive sweating beyond the physiological needs of the body (Solish et al. 2005), with a prevalence of 2.8% in the United States of America (USA) (Strutton et al. 2004), 9.3% in Germany (for focal hyperhidrosis) (Augustin et al. 2013) and 2.79–5.75% in Japan (Fujimoto et al. 2013). Most patients experience hyperhidrosis in more than one body site

P. Kamudoni et al., *Living with Chronic Disease: Measuring Important Patient-Reported Outcomes*, https://doi.org/10.1007/978-981-10-8414-0_3

and the most prevalent sites are palmoplantar, axillar or generalised (Liu et al. 2016; Augustin et al. 2013). Studies from Germany, Brazil and Japan have reported that 30–37.9% of patients with hyperhidrosis are frequently or constantly bothered by their sweating, resulting in impairment in daily activities, in psychological well-being and in study or work (Augustin et al. 2013; Fujimoto et al. 2013; Lima et al. 2015).

The clinical management of hyperhidrosis depends on its severity and location. Clinical severity assessment utilises measures including gravimetry, minor's iodine test and evaporimetry. Unlike other dermatological conditions, hyperhidrosis is poorly treated, with only 35% visiting a doctor (Strutton et al. 2004). Nonetheless, even those seeking treatment face a hard choice between expensive treatments such as Botox, high-risk surgical interventions such as ETS surgery or other much cheaper but less effective treatments. Consequently, the majority of patients survive with an unmanaged condition. In the long term, this poses a real risk of patients developing psychological sequelae owning to the persistent impact.

Gravimetric assessment quantifies the amount of sweat produced over a particular skin area, within a given time period, by use of a filter paper and a microbalance (Hund et al. 2002). The paper is weighed before and after its application to a thoroughly cleaned affected skin area, over a given time. Weight per unit of time can then be calculated from the before-and-after weight measurements. Kalkan et al. (1998) applied a modification of this method in palmar hyperhidrosis. A padded glove made from gauze material was used in place of the filter paper, and surgical gloves were worn on top to prevent moisture from escaping. The weighing then uses an electronic scale with sensitivity of 0.0001 g. The minor's iodine test is used in demarcating the area affected by hyperhidrosis (Glogau 2001). The affected area is wiped with an iodine tincture, and then a starch is applied after thorough drying. New sweat secreted leads to a colour change demarcating the area affected, following the reaction between the iodine molecule and the starch. Assessment may be facilitated by taking a digital photo. The ventilation capsule method assesses sweat production based on moisture evaporating from the skin measured using an electronic device (skin moisture meter) (Keller et al. 2009). A cup of 1 cm diameter connected to the device is used to capture moisture leaving the skin, with the amount of sweating over time (e.g. mg/cm/minute) read off a digital sweat meter reading (Ohhashi et al. 1998).

Clinical measures may have, however, limited usefulness in the management of hyperhidrosis for a variety of reasons. First, their anticipated objectivity is questionable. Cut-off quantity of sweat between patients and non-patients is unclear, an artefact of intra-individual variation of sweat production at different times and situations (Hund et al. 2002). Currently suggested cut-off values of 50 mg/5 min for females and 100 mg/5 min for males are arbitrary, and their specificity or sensitivity has not been established (Hornberger et al. 2004). The other issue relates to the practicality of these measures. The cumbersome nature of these clinical tests makes them challenging to apply in routine clinical practice, limiting their usefulness to a few cases and research settings. The assessment of quality of life impairment resulting from the sweating, therefore, is important to the diagnosis and management of hyperhidrosis in routine practice. A disease model for hyperhidrosis is presented in Fig. 3.1.

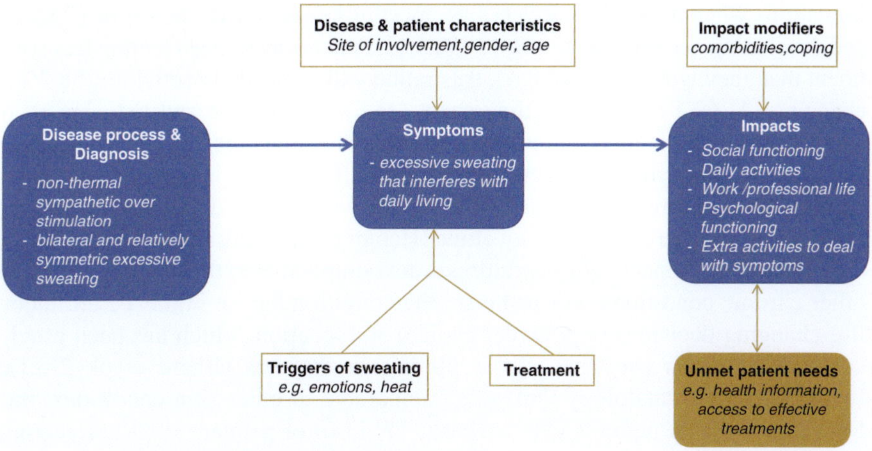

Fig. 3.1 Disease conceptual model for hyperhidrosis

Impact on HRQoL

The overall nature and extent of the handicap and impairment in the patient's life resulting from skin disease is well understood (Jowett and Ryan 1985; Finlay and Ryan 1996). Its impact extends across various areas of life (such as emotional distress, impact on social life such as in relationships, professional life, physical discomfort from itching or wet skin, and the burden associated with managing the condition). This also has to be seen in the light of skin's high visibility as well as its particular role in self-image (Beltraminelli and Itin 2008). On the other hand, for conditions such as hyperhidrosis, the laboratory-clinical measures of sweat are difficult to interpret, apart from reliability and practicality issues (Hund et al. 2002), leaving self-reported impacts on the patient's life as a 'vital sign' of disease activity (Chren 2005), especially in routine clinical practice.

The current evidence on the impairment in daily life activities and HRQoL in hyperhidrosis is based on standardised HRQoL instruments and self-reported disease severity scales such as the HDSS or the DLQI; one qualitative study is also available. Overall quality of life of patients is reduced as a result of the condition. Scores of the dermatology life quality index (DLQI) ranged from 10 to 14 for axillary hyperhidrosis, 8.8–15 for palmar hyperhidrosis, 13 for craniofacial hyperhidrosis and 9.4 for the trunk across 14 studies in hyperhidrosis patients (Lupin et al. 2014; Rosell et al. 2012; Muller et al. 2012; Kim et al. 2010; Campanati et al. 2010; Amini et al. 2008; Bechara et al. 2007; Hamm et al. 2006; Solish et al. 2005; Innocenzi et al. 2005; Campanati et al. 2003; Tan and Solish 2002; Swartling et al. 2001).

Patients have previously also reported feeling that their life is taken over by hyperhidrosis (Thomas et al. 2006). For example, aspects of daily living including choice of clothing and relationships with family and friends have been reported to be affected (Thomas et al. 2006). In a study by Solish (2006), respondents reported limitations when in public places (74%), meeting people for the first time (70.2%) and developing personal relationships (58.5%). Patients mentioned feeling less confident than they would like (69.8%), frustration with some daily activities (58.2%), changing (41.6%) or reducing time spent (34.6%) on leisure and reducing time spent working. Patients reported being emotionally impaired (74%), having less confidence (74%), reduced work performance (63%) and influences on career choice (42%), whereas a comparative control group registered no impairment in a study based at a German university clinic (Hamm et al. 2006).

The HRQoL impacts of hyperhidrosis are comparable to those experienced in other chronic conditions. For instance, the condition has an influence on major life-changing decisions (e.g. career choice) and location, which has been previously observed in psoriasis, cystic fibrosis or diabetes (Bhatti et al. 2011). Impairment in dermatology QoL was comparable to other skin conditions: the DLQI scores from patients with axillary (17–11.6) or palmar (18–9.1) hyperhidrosis were comparable to, or worse than, those from patients with dermatitis (inpatient) (16.2) or psoriasis (13.9). Cina and Clase (1999) found the lifestyle intrusiveness associated with hyperhidrosis to be worse than in other known chronic conditions, such as end-stage renal disease, rheumatoid arthritis or multiple sclerosis.

As a long-term condition, non-surgical treatments in hyperhidrosis are largely concerned with enhancing the patients' HRQoL and well-being: their ability to manage everyday routine such as performing housework, interacting with others, participating and contributing to social activity and performance at work/school. On the other hand, treatment therapies in hyperhidrosis are often associated with unbearable side effects such as compensatory sweating (ETS surgery, inter-dermal Botox injection), mouth dryness (anticholinergics) or transient hand weakness (inter-dermal Botox injection), raising the question of whether benefits of treatment outweigh the burden associated with side effects. Patient-reported symptomatic adverse effects of treatments are poorly understood in hyperhidrosis. The assessment of PROs such as HRQoL and patient-reported symptomatic AEs of treatment may offer a comprehensive framework for a more holistic evaluation of drug benefits and risk for the individual patient.

The burden on a patient's daily life associated with skin disease is profound, often exceeding that of various chronic diseases conditions (Finlay 1998; Basra and Shahrukh 2009). It is unclear why HRQoL impairment is worse in hyperhidrosis in comparison to other conditions such as psoriasis as noted by Hamm and colleagues (Hamm et al. 2006). Several explanations are plausible. First, patients with hyperhidrosis report feeling their life as being taken over by hyperhidrosis all the time. This reflects the persistence (and frequency) of sweating episodes and their related impacts. Sweating episodes are accompanied by feelings of anxiety (besides other negative emotions), in a chicken-egg circle. Patients get anxious that they may sweat and in turn more anxiety leads to more sweating. This is consistent with earlier views on the disease, where psychiatric underpinnings were suspected (chicken-egg) (Ruchinskas 2007). This is also consistent with the view of hyperhidrosis as a multifactorial condition (Beltraminelli and Itin 2008). The greater impact on QOL in this case is being alluded to by the strong feedback between the psychiatric impacts and sweating.

Part II: The Qualitative Development of the Hyperhidrosis Quality of Life Index (HidroQoL)

Drug regulatory authorities such as the FDA require documentation on the process followed in the development of PRO instruments used in making labelling claims, as evidence for content validity (US FDA 2009). This points towards the need for an organised and well-thought-out development process as described in the roadmap presented in Chap. 2. The early stages of the process involve setting the objectives and broad research strategy, generating hypothesis about the concepts, gathering and selecting item concepts and then designing and building the measure. These aspects are illustrated in the current chapter using an example from some of our research in hyperhidrosis.

Humanistic aspects of disease burden reflect issues that are of most relevance to patients, their families and society at large and thus are an important element of the overall burden of disease. As the patient is the expert in their experience with a condition, their voice should matter most when considering such outcomes. Qualitative research methods are quite useful for obtaining insights into the beliefs, values and perceptions of informants captured in their own words (Pope and Mays 2008). This would offer key insights into factors confounding patient outcomes, the long-term consequences of impairment and how patients deal with the condition. In addition to qualitative interviews with patients, a structured literature review and expert input are useful sources of evidence supporting the early stages of PRO measure development.

Step 1: Define Objectives of Development of the PROM

Broad Aim

To conceptualise, develop and validate a disease-specific instrument for assessing HRQoL in hyperhidrosis that would be applicable in clinical research as well as routine clinical practice.

Secondary Objectives

1. To explore the experiences of patients with hyperhidrosis in order to obtain an in-depth understanding of the extent and nature of QoL impacts.
2. To create a conceptual framework for HRQoL in hyperhidrosis.
3. To develop a disease-specific instrument for evaluating QoL impacts in hyperhidrosis based on the experiences of patients.
4. To assess whether the content of the new disease-specific instrument was relevant to patients with hyperhidrosis; adequate and appropriate for measuring the concept of quality of life.
5. To establish the dimensional structure of the new instrument and to perform item reduction.
6. To assess the reliability and the construct validity of the new instrument.
7. To establish the minimum important clinical difference (MCID) value of the new instrument.

Step 2: Hypothesis Generation and Conceptualisation

The initial steps in the development of the HidroQoL involved a literature review to uncover the impacts of hyperhidrosis on the patient, a critical appraisal of PRO measures used in hyperhidrosis and a qualitative study in patients with hyperhidrosis to capture patient's experience with hyperhidrosis. A structured literature review was instrumental to the initial understanding of core impacts/HRQOL issues important to patients with hyperhidrosis and how these are perceived and described by the patient. Apart from providing a rationale for assessing HRQoL, this provided an important foundation for the development of a new PRO measure for assessing QoL impacts of hyperhidrosis. In addition, critical appraisal of PRO instruments used in hyperhidrosis was performed to determine if any of the existing instruments was fit for purpose or alternatively to understand the gaps and limitations with current measures. This led to a clear rationale for developing a new PRO measure focusing on HRQoL, and provided evidence to generate initial conceptual framework for the measure, and subsequently the relevant content was generated through qualitative research.

Methods

Literature Review to Uncover the Impacts of Hyperhidrosis on Patients' HRQoL

The literature searches were carried out in multiple bibliographic databases including PubMed, Google Scholar, Ovid/Embase and Scopus. A combination of three blocks of terms was applied to the title, abstract and keywords of the databases: block 1, *hyperhidrosis*; block 2, *effects, effects on patients, impact and impact on patients*; and block 3, *health-related quality of life, quality of life, patient's life, daily life, everyday life and lifestyle*. For searches in PubMed, using MeSH term would be recommended. The initial eligibility criteria were that studies should be investigating QOL in patients with primary hyperhidrosis using qualitative research methods. When only one relevant study was found, eligibility criteria were changed to include studies that had employed quantitative methods. A structured process was followed in sourcing and selecting studies for inclusion in the review.

Critical Appraisal of the Instruments Used in HRQoL Measurement in Hyperhidrosis

To identify instruments that have been used in HRQoL assessment in hyperhidrosis, a literature search was carried out in PubMed, PsycINFO and Embase. The initial search was based on the following terms: 'hyperhidrosis and quality of life', 'hyperhidrosis and daily life', 'hyperhidrosis and clinical trial' and 'hyperhidrosis and impact'. References in the papers initially extracted were also searched to identify more material for our review. An additional search strategy was based on the identified instruments, e.g. 'SF-36 and hyperhidrosis' and 'DLQI and hyperhidrosis', to identify all studies using the instruments in hyperhidrosis patients. A study was included if it reported the measurement of HRQoL in hyperhidrosis patients using a

HRQoL instrument or if it reported the psychometric properties of such an instrument. An instrument was included if it was developed for the measurement of HRQoL and if it had been used in hyperhidrosis patients. Such instruments could be disease-specific, dermatology-specific or generic. We limited ourselves to HRQoL self-assessed by patients, either self-completed questionnaire or interviewer administered. Study-specific instruments were excluded.

Psychometric information and descriptive details related to instruments were extracted and reviewed according to standard quality criteria for HRQoL instruments (Lohr 2002; Both et al. 2007). Attributes considered included content validity, construct validity, convergence validity, internal consistency, test-retest reliability, responsiveness, floor/ceiling effects, interpretability and minimal clinically important differences. Ultimately, the appraisal was intended at assessing the appropriateness of HRQOL measures (content relevance) as well as fitness for purpose (measurement attributes).

Results

Impacts of Hyperhidrosis on Patients' HRQoL

Thomas et al. (2006) investigated lifestyle impact, compensating behaviours and treatment experiences of female hyperhidrosis patients, through three focus group discussions with 21 female patients with hyperhidrosis from the US. Patients were recruited through the database of the international hyperhidrosis society (IHHS). Patients reported effects on their relationships with family and friends, and in their professional interactions. Additionally, effects were reported on patient's self-confidence and self-esteem, besides the psychological distress. Patients mentioned feeling their life was taken over by the hyperhidrosis all the time. They worried about their clothes getting soiled which led embarrassment when it happened. One participant was quoted as follows:

> we were running around...I had to put my shirt around my waist because I had a spot on the back of my pants from the waist down to the knees. It looked like I wet myself and I didn't want people to make fun of me on the last day of school.

Patients reported on the inconvenience, effort and cost associated with strategies employed to deal with the sweating and its symptoms, for example, choosing clothing that hid the sweat, using tissues and pads and using a fan when getting dressed. While this study provides valuable insights, exclusion of males means that gender-specific experiences of males were not reflected in the results. On the other hand, there is no indication whether the issues of relevance to patients had been exhaustively explored.

Tools Used in HRQoL Measurement in Hyperhidrosis Patients

Fourteen instruments have been applied in assessing HRQoL in hyperhidrosis; this includes four generic instruments, four dermatology-specific instruments and five hyperhidrosis-specific instruments. The basic description and psychometric properties of the measures are presented in Table 3.1.

Table 3.1 Psychometric properties of PRO measures in hyperhidrosis

Questionnaire	Content validity	Construct validity	Convergent validity	Internal consistency	Test-retest reliability	Responsiveness	Floor and ceiling effects	Interpretability	MCID	Respondent burden	Structure
Disease specific HRQol instruments											
HHIQ[1,2,3]	++	++	++	++	0	0	++	0	0	0	0
HDSS[4,5,6,7]	++	++	++	na	++	++	0	+	+	++	na
HS[8,9]	++	++	+	++	0	++	0	+	0	0	na
HQ[10]	++	+	0	++	0	0	0	0	0	++	+
HQLQ[11,12,13]	–	–	0	0	0	–	0	0	0	0	0
AMIR[14]	++	+	0	++	0	0	–	0	0	0	+
Dermatology HRQol-specific questionnaire											
FLQA[15,16]	++	++	+	+	++	++	+	++	0	0	0
DLQI[17,18,19]	++	++	++	++	+	++	+	++	++	++	–
Skindex[20,21,22,23,24,25]	++	++	++	++	++	++	++	++	0	+	+
PBI[26,27,28]	++	++	+	++	+	+	+	+	0	0	+
Generic HRQol questionnaire											
SF-36[29, 30]	++	++	++	++	++	++	+	+	++	+	+
SF-12[30]	++	++	++	++	++	+	++	+		++	+
NHP[24, 30]	++	++	++	+	++	+	+	0	0	++	+
IIRS[31,32,33]	+	++	++	++	++	++	0	0	0	0	+

Note: Although Teale, Roberts et al. (2002) claim that the HHIQ has favourable internal consistency, test-retest reliability and construct and convergent validity, the relevant correlations were not reported

References: (1) Teale, Roberts et al. (2002); (2) Naumann, Hamm et al. (2002); (3) Jonathan, Nina et al. (2004); (4) Lowe, Campanati et al. (2004); (5) David, Jonathan et al. (2004); (6) Solish, Benohanian et al. (2005); (7) Solish, Bertucci et al. (2007); (8) Keller et al. (2009); (9) Keller, Sekons et al. (2001); (10) Kuo et al. (2004); (11) Panhofer, Zacherl et al. (2006); (12) de Campos, Kauffman et al. (2003); (13) Ambrogi, Campione et al. (2009); (14) Amir et al. (2000); (15) Augustin, Zschocke et al. (2000); (16) Augustin, Lange et al. (2004); (17) Finlay and Khan (1994); (18) Basra, Fenech et al. (2008); (19) Kowalski (2007); (20) Chren, Lasek et al. (1996);(21) Augustin, Wenninger et al. (2004); (22) Abeni, Picardi et al. (2002); (23) Nijsten, Sampogna et al. (2006); (24) Both, Essink-Bot et al. (2007); (25) Prinsen, Lindeboom et al. (2010); (26) Augustin, Radtke et al. (2009); (27) Augustin, Reich et al. (2008); (28) Blome, Augustin et al. (2011); (29) Both et al. (2007); (30) McDowell (2006); (31) Devins, Binik et al. (1983); (32) Cinà and Clase (1999); (33) Bieling, Rowa et al. (2001)

Among the skin-specific measures, only the DLQI and the PBI instruments had been validated in hyperhidrosis patients. These measures are overall more relevant for hyperhidrosis patients in comparison to generic measures. Given the DLQI's brevity, simpler scoring system and availability of cut-offs for clinical significance (in the form of MID) for hyperhidrosis, it would be the preferred of the two.

Of the disease-specific measures found, the HDSS and the HHIQ were the most validated. Although the HDSS has been included in this review and has also been used in other trials as a measure of QoL, it is strictly a measure of disease severity and interference of hyperhidrosis in everyday life. Moreover, as a single item instrument, it does not provide a detailed picture of QOL, and its four-level scoring might not have much scope for capturing changes in patient's condition over time. On the other hand, while the HHIQ is indeed promising both in terms of coverage issues relevant to patients, it was not designed for use in routine clinical practice; its internal structure has not been tested, it has no scoring system, and no information has been provided for interpretation of scores. All disease-specific measures lacked evidence of temporal stability (i.e. test-retest reliability). Evidence of construct validity and responsiveness was not based on robust approaches. For example, only factor analysis exploring factorial structure has been undertaken in one measure only (hyperhidrosis questionnaire).

Among the generic measures, only the IIRS had been validated in hyperhidrosis patients (Cinà and Clase 1999). Other generic HRQoL measures such as the SF-36 were seen to include items irrelevant for hyperhidrosis while omitting key issues relevant in this patient population. This also applies to dermatology-specific measures though to a lesser degree. Moreover, except for the Patient Benefit Index (PBI), the other measures have not been validated in this patient population.

In the studies reviewed, HRQOL impairment in hyperhidrosis alluded to social functioning and emotional role limitation, whereas dermatology-specific impacts were related to daily activities, personal relationships and symptoms and feelings. The necessity for more showers; sweating after consumption of alcohol, spicy foods or coffee; and facing a limited choice of clothing represent disruptions in patients' lives.

This review has revealed a deficit in the current measurement of HRQOL in hyperhidrosis. There is need for a new measure which would assess HRQOL specific to patients with hyperhidrosis, with its content underpinned by patient experiences and quality of life issues they face, with demonstrated optimal psychometric attributes of construct validity, inter-temporal stability, internally consistent, tested internal structure and unidimensional scales. In order to ensure clinical feasibility of such a measure, adequate attention would have to be given to ensure its practicality, for example, having a small number of questions as much as possible to allow all questions to fit on one side of an A4 page and using a simple scoring procedure.

Step 3: Qualitative Method to Understand Patient's Experience

Methods

A mix of qualitative methods including interviews, focus groups and online surveys for data collection was used to investigate the impact of hyperhidrosis on QoL of individuals with hyperhidrosis. Study participants included members of hyperhidrosis patient support groups including the *UK Hyperhidrosis Patient Support Group*, the *Very Sweaty Betty* and other groups on *Facebook*; all of these also had online communities. Inclusion criteria included ≥16 years old, self-reported hyperhidrosis, seeking treatment and able to communicate in English. Exclusion criteria included excessive sweating related to a particular health issue, based on late onset of sweating and the presence of comorbidities/use of medication known to be associated with sweating.

Ethics approval for this study was obtained from the ethics committee of the University Hospital of Greifswald, Germany. Informed consent was obtained from all participants before their participation in the focus group discussion, interviews and electronically for survey participants. Purposive sampling and snow-ball sampling were used in order to ensure the inclusion of patients with all types of hyperhidrosis, such as those affected in different body areas or with different demographic characteristics. Snow-ball sampling was quite natural to recruitment using social media and took advantage of individuals' typical usage of social media (e.g. Facebook).

In the focus groups/interviews, participants were invited to share their experience of living with hyperhidrosis. The participants were prompted to explain their responses, for instance, by providing examples. The interviewer/moderator also raised questions in relation to specific areas of life known to be heavily impacted by hyperhidrosis and overlooked by the patients.

Online surveys were developed based on the results of the focus group discussion and interviews and included open-ended questions. A link to the surveys was posted on the portal for the UK hyperhidrosis society and other forums. Interviews were tape-recorded then transcribed verbatim. The focus group discussions and open surveys were already in text format. Applying a grounded theory approach (Bowen 2006), transcripts of data were analysed to identify key themes and concepts. As a data-driven methodology, the analysis followed an inductive process, with the concepts and structure emerging/extracted from the data. No a priori hypotheses were imposed on the data. In practice, the analysis involved a continuous circle of studying the primary data, and developing interpretations and concepts, with additional data, and earlier interpretations were revisited and further developed.

A researcher coded the data using NVIVO 9 software (QSR International). Initially, a codebook was developed based on the initial data transcripts; this was then discussed with the research team before all the data were coded. The initial codebook evolved as more data were analysed. The coding process involved first identifying and coding issues from the data (low level coding), then identifying similar concepts based on the low level codes and organising these into subthemes and themes (Braun and Clarke 2006). Further insights into the data were sought by comparing themes across different hyperhidrosis sites or demographic factors.

Findings

Qualitative Method to Understand Patient's Experience

Seventy-one patients took part in the study (*n* = 9 for focus groups; *n* = 32 for semi-structured interviews; and *n* = 30 for online surveys), out of an initial 100 individuals recruited. The mean age of participants (males = 21, female = 50) was 35 years (range 16–67) and the mean duration of hyperhidrosis was 23 years (3–60 years). Participants reporting generalised hyperhidrosis comprised 28% of the sample and were the largest group.

Theme saturation occurred on the 33rd patients, i.e. no new themes emerged after this point. Seventeen themes within seven major topics/areas including daily life (reported by 95.8% of participants), psychological life (91.5%), social life (90.1%), professional life (74.6%), dealing with the condition (74.6%), unmet health care needs (64.8%) and physical impact (53.5%) were identified from the data. This can be summarised as follows:

- *Daily life* such as hobbies, everyday activities including using touch technologies and lifestyle, e.g. choice of clothing and food/drink, were affected.
- Impacts related to *psychological well-being* included negative emotions, fear of people's reaction, self-image, feeling restricted and loss of control.
- Social life was affected in terms of not being able to be in social situations, having physical contact and personal relationships and intimacy.
- *Managing the condition* represented additional burden for patients, e.g. personal hygiene and special chores, time spent and financial burden in managing the condition.
- *Physical impacts* reported included physical discomfort, secondary skin problems and body odour.
- *Unmet healthcare needs* mentioned by the patients included the clinical management of condition and lack of information.
- Professional/school life was reported as work/school tasks and career.

A selection of quotations from the patients are presented in the Appendix. Full results from this phase of work are published elsewhere (Kamudoni et al. 2017).

Insights into Themes

The findings demonstrate that the impact of hyperhidrosis on the lives of the patients is broad, affecting all areas of life such as daily life, psychological well-being, social life, professional life, dealing with the condition, unmet healthcare needs and physical impact, with psychosocial issues playing a central role. Negative emotions such as anxiety and embarrassment were often highlighted as a reason for avoiding various activities, resulting in handicap in basic daily activities. For example, shopping and paying for groceries were challenging partly because patients were uncomfortable with being near others or did not want to brush hands with the cashier. Having wet palms and negative emotions was an underlying issue in impacts on professional life.

On the extreme, the participants often resorted to avoidance of situations that would aggravate the sweating or the impacts; this may in turn have long-term or major consequences such as affecting major life-changing decision or personality change.

The importance of psychosocial impacts may be further amplified by the multifactorial nature of hyperhidrosis—excessive sweating symptoms are exacerbated by patient's psychological response such as negative emotions (Beltraminelli and Itin 2008). It has been shown empirically that anxiety or stress and being in social situations are more important aggravating factors for hyperhidrosis than heat or summer season (Park et al. 2010). This reflects the perennial nature of hyperhidrosis.

No major differences were noted in areas of impact such as choice of clothing, fear of leaving sweat marks on objects, impacts on social life, impacts on emotional life, career choices and hobbies. Even in aspects such as the burden of dealing with the condition, although the exact tools used were different across different hyperhidrosis sites, the burden that these represented for the patients was similar.

Furthermore, the current findings suggest that individuals with hyperhidrosis have healthcare needs that are currently not being met, such as access to treatment, adequacy of patient information and support in dealing with the psychological scourge of hyperhidrosis. Similar information problems have been noted in other dermatologic conditions such as psoriasis (Golics et al. 2009). This suggests that individuals with skin disorders including hyperhidrosis may benefit from interventions helping them deal with the wider impacts of their condition such as counselling, education and psychotherapy, accessible within and outside the clinic. In this context, online platforms may offer a wide scope for increasing the availability of such services. A previous study reported that individuals with hyperhidrosis spend 15–60 min a day in managing symptoms of the condition and that 50–70% change their clothes more than twice a day (Hamm et al. 2006). One in every five patients relies on some form of accessory to manage their daily life normally (Strutton et al. 2004). A good part of dealing with the condition involves disguising or concealing the sweating.

Step 4: Design and Build PRO Measure

This section illustrates the process of developing of a conceptual framework and drafting of items/content for a PRO using the HidroQoL. The conceptual framework clearly defines the concept being measured, the rationale for undertaking the measurement, the target population, as well as the context of measurement (DeVellis 2016). Skipping this critical step may have consequences for the clarity of the dimensional structure, may complicate subsequent data analysis and may ultimately obscure interpretation of scale scores (Rothman et al. 2007).

Generating the Initial Items for the New PRO Measure

Following content analysis of the data collected through interviews, focus groups and open surveys with hyperhidrosis patients (Steps 2 and 3), major HRQoL issues were identified. An instrument drafting summit was organised where a team including PRO experts, pharmacists and clinicians developed/drafted the new PRO measure. In addition, two patients were also consulted during the process, to obtain their views and feedback on the drafted items.

HRQoL themes and subthemes were selected for inclusion based on various a priori criteria (DeVellis 2016; Patrick et al. 2011a). Issues with a prevalence of 5% or more in the qualitative sample were included; age- or gender-specific issues, regardless of being mentioned by less than 5% of the sample, were also included. The team aimed at drafting the items to be concise and simple with a maximum of six words or less; each item was to represent a single concept, based on language used by the patients, and free of technical jargon (Streiner and Norman 2008). The first prototype instrument included 75 items and was scored on a 6-point Likert scale (Appendix—Fig. 3.2).

Choosing a Response Format

Once the items were drafted, an appropriate response categorisation, fitting to each item stem, the underlying target concept(s), recall period and the mode of administration was crafted. Initially, a 7-point Likert scale was considered for the first prototype questionnaire applying different descriptors for each item. This was subsequently thought to be cumbersome and was therefore revised during the developmental process to a 5-point Likert scale (~ plus a 'not relevant' option); descriptors were common for all items. This was seen to strike a balance between applicability and need to offer sufficient choice and precision.

The decision regarding the most relevant response scaling involved consideration of various options. For example, although visual analogue scales (VAS) were thought to offer a wide range over which patients could choose from, this was considered to be unnecessary and thought to add undue burden on respondents and with that a risk for score variation unrelated to the underlying condition. The optimal maximum number of options on a response categorisation system is suggested to be around 7 (±2), based on the maximum number of categories that people are capable of distinguishing (Streiner and Norman 2008). On the other hand, offering far less than the optimal number of options, e.g. yes or no option, is not recommended, due to the threat of losing information.

Choosing a Frame of Reference

Further, the period of time respondents needed to consider in producing answers, the recall period, was set. In turn, the wording of the items and responses and instructions would reflect this decision. The suitability of the recall period depends on measurement goals, for instance, long-term impacts versus efficacy of intervention; the nature of the construct, symptoms or HRQoL impacts; frequency of assessments; and, ultimately, the target population (Norquist et al. 2011). The shortest recall period feasible is recommended. A recall period that is too short may unnecessarily overburden the respondent; on the other hand exceeding 1 month may be associated with increased recall bias (Frost et al. 2007a). 'At present' was chosen as recall period for the new instrument. Responses based on the condition of the respondents during the time of assessment would be subject to minimal recall bias as the respondents would produce answers spontaneously, minimising noise in the measurement process.

Choosing a Mode of Administration

The choice of how the instrument will be applied during data collection, whether in-person interview, telephone, paper and pencil, electronic or web-based, tends to have an influence on data obtained (Streiner and Norman 2008; Frost et al. 2007a). Suitability of the mode depends on a number of factors such as the preferences of the target participants and the construct under assessment, the content of the instrument for instance recall period and the number and frequency of assessments, among others (DeVellis 2016). Paper-and-pencil administration was chosen for the new instrument because of its ease of administration, making it easy and practical for routine clinical practice while avoiding 'social desirability' issues salient in modes such as in-person interview. Furthermore, to reach patient populations outside the clinic, it would also be administered via the Internet, which may allow coverage of patients outside the clinic; besides there were other advantages, for instance, a stronger sense of anonymity for respondents.

Choosing a Structure and Format

The structure of the instrument, including its formatting, is an important element of the instrument, with impacts on the accuracy and reliability of data collected (Haynes et al. 1995). For example, formatting has potential implications on navigational errors (such as item non-response and misinterpretation) and respondent and administrative burden (Mullin et al. 2000). In order to ensure a simple, clear, consistent and natural design, the following decisions were taken:

- Items containing similar content were grouped together.
- A light grey shading of 0.4 cm thickness was used to separate items, in order to reflect the responses that related to a particular item; grid lines were avoided.
- Tick boxes were provided for giving responses.
- Response categories followed a natural ordering from 'no, not at all' on the extreme left to 'very much' on the extreme right.
- Instructions were provided on what was being measured and the relevant recall period for participants to use in recalling their answers and how to choose responses. Instructions presented on the first page were circumscribed in a border to enhance their visibility. Instructions were also included on each page throughout the instrument.

The earliest prototype of the new questionnaire contained a total of 75 HRQoL issues (Appendix—Fig. 3.2). Subsequently this was reorganised to form the 47-item HidroQoL mostly by combining similar issues. Its items were scored on a 5-point Likert scale with an additional 'not applicable' option.

Concluding Remarks

In this chapter, we have described an example, based on research in hyperhidrosis, illustrating how the first three steps of the roadmap presented in Chap. 2—item gathering, item selection and building the tool—might be implemented. The evidence on the impacts of hyperhidrosis on the patient's life gathered through the literature review indicated substantive impairment in all areas of HRQoL, with social life impacts being central. Reduction in dermatology-specific HRQoL was comparable or worse than that in other dermatologic diseases such as psoriasis and rosacea. The literature review also identified a total of 13 instruments, previously used in hyperhidrosis to assess HRQoL or symptoms including disease-specific, dermatology-specific as well as generic instruments. A gap analysis of the measures revealed various limitations such as lack of content validity in hyperhidrosis, inadequate basic psychometric properties, lack of practicality, applicability and clinical appropriateness.

The use of qualitative methods has provided deep insights into the major issues influencing the HRQoL of patients with hyperhidrosis. Further, the unmet healthcare needs of relevance to the patients' HRQoL were also identified, including treatment- and information-related issues. The HRQoL issues identified from the qualitative study, which are based on the patient's own words, provided a rich source for developing the content of a novel hyperhidrosis-specific QoL questionnaire for assessing QoL impacts of hyperhidrosis, ensuring that the new measure was indeed appropriate and had the right emphasis for the target patient population. The structured process followed in the development of the new instrument, including the development of a conceptual framework, having a clear criteria for the content and subsequently drafting the content of the instrument in line with the criteria, further enhanced the appropriateness and suitability of the new measure for hyperhidrosis patients.

The new instrument was intended for assessing impacts of QoL of individual patients in routine clinical practice and in clinical research. The target patient population includes all forms of hyperhidrosis, based on body area affected. The construct was being measured at a level generic enough for the items to have relevance to all forms of hyperhidrosis. The items reflected aspects of QoL affected by hyperhidrosis based on the personal feelings and perceptions of the patients. Response categorization was chosen to reflect different levels of impairment in the concepts addressed in each item. Instructions were written to be clear, highly visible and offer useful guide to the patients in the questionnaire completion process. Timeframe of reference was chosen to minimise recall bias and match the aspects of hyperhidrosis QoL. Formatting decisions were made to realise a simple, natural and organised design ensuring easy navigation and minimal respondent burden and provide an attractive questionnaire.

The data collection in case study benefited from triangulation of several qualitative data collection methods including focus groups, semi-structured interviews and online open surveys. During the focus group discussions, interactions among participants helped with stimulating new aspects or topics of discussion, generating additional data otherwise not realisable (Patrick et al. 2011b). The interviews, on the other hand, provided in-depth and detailed information about an individual's experience besides the relative ease of arranging appointments with the patients (Patrick et al. 2011b). The surveys with open-ended questions were the low-hanging fruit, as they could be implemented with relative ease, while providing a good balance between ability to reach large numbers of patients relatively easily while still allowing respondents to give detailed description of their opinions (Bowling 2009). However, lack of opportunity for probing as is the case in focus group discussions or interviews may limit the depth of information provided.

The implications of the approach taken were multifold. First, it ensured that the instrument being developed had high applicability for the intended measurement purpose and acceptability in the target patient population (patients with hyperhidrosis). Second, the involvement of the target patient population in item elicitation was essential to the content validity of the new measure (Rothman et al. 2009). Ultimately, this reflects the essence and nature of measures of QoL impact as a vehicle for patients to express their voice in relation to the impacts of their condition on all aspects of daily life (Basra and Shahrukh 2009).

Appendix

1 Sweating influences my choice of clothing (e.g. design, colour or material)

2 I avoid exposing soaked clothing around the armpits area sweating (e.g. I avoid raising my arms)

3 I do activities at a slower pace due to the sweating (e.g. physical activities such as walking)

4 Sweating influences my choice of footwear

5 Holidays are less enjoyable because of sweating

6 I have trouble handling money with my hands because of the sweating

7 I have trouble giving care to children because of my sweating

8 I avoid certain foods e.g. spicy foods because they make me sweat (gustatory sweating)

9 I find it difficult to do hobbiesthat involve physical activities (e.g.walking, cycling,exercising, playing musical instruments)

10 Doing work-related activities is difficult (e.g. dealing with clients, caring for patients, working with tools)

11 Sweating restricts my life (e.g. stops me from travelling)

12 Sweating influences my career decisions (e.g. choice of work)

13 Handling paper documents and writing is difficult because of my sweating

14 I avoid outdoor activities (sun-basking or gardening)

15 I have trouble using hand operated electronics due to my sweating (e.g. computer keyboards, cell-phone, touch-screens)

16 My sweating makes shopping difficult

17 Activities involving walking barefoot are difficult because of my sweating

Fig. 3.2 Prototype PRO measure v1

18 I dread holding or shaking hands with others

19 Sweating interferes with my personal relationships (e.g. with friends or partner)

20 I feel embarrassed because of the sweating

21 I can’t socialize as much as I would like to

22 I am afraid of meeting new people

23 I fear speaking to groups of people because of my sweating (e.g. doing presentations, meetings, interviews)

24 I avoid going out (e.g. to parties, eating in restaurants)

25 I am a virtual recluse because of my sweating

26 I can't find a treatment that works for me

27 My doctor does not understand my condition

28 Adapting to the sweating is difficult (e.g. maintaining body hygiene, need to keep fan or air condition on)

29 I disguise my sweating (e.g. wear gloves, jacket, socks)

30 I carry spare clothes or towel with me because of my sweating

31 I fear that my sweating will be noticed by others

32 I look untidy

33 I change clothes...

34 I shower…

35 I feel less attractive

36 I can't wear a hairstyle or make-up of my choice

37 Sweating makes me feel nervous

38 Sweating has taken overmy life

39 I fear doing new things because of my sweating

40 I feel hopeless

41 My sweating makes me feel sad

42 I feel miserable because of my sweating

Fig. 3.2 (continued)

43 I dread summers because of the sweating

44 I fear that my sweating is worsening

45 I think about sweating ...

46 My self-esteem is low because of my sweating

47 I feel less confident because of my sweating

48 I am emotionally drained because of the sweating

49 I feel more self-conscious because of my sweating

50 Sweating makes my sexual life less enjoyable

51 I fear leaving sweat marks on objects

52 I have trouble being in crowded spaces because of my sweating (e.g. in bus or train)

53 I am drenched in sweat (e.g. my clothes are wet)

54 My sweating is physically uncomfortable

55 Light movements make me sweat (e.g. getting dressed)

56 I slide in and out of my shoes

57 Sweat gets into my eyes

58 My feet give an unpleasant odour

59 It is difficult to grip objects in my hands because of my sweating (e.g. tools, door knobs)

60 I am afraid to physically express affection because of my sweating (hugging and cuddling)

61 I avoid getting close to people (when sitting, queing, dancing)

62 I feel that others judge me because of my sweating

63 I feel depressed because of my sweating

64 I fear rejection from others because of my sweating

65 My sweating makes housework difficult (e.g. cleaning, cooking)

66 My sweating exerts a financial burden on my life

67 Casual walking makes me sweat

68 Myskin is sore and cracked because of my sweating

69 I can't do things spontaneously

70 Sweating makes driving difficult

Fig. 3.2 (continued)

71 Doing physical activities is difficult because of my sweating (e.g. manual work)

72 My body (or clothes) gives a bad odour because of the sweating

73 I sweat even in winter

74 I get other skin problems as a result of my sweating

75 I feel hot even in winter

Fig. 3.2 (continued)

References

Amini M, Harmsze AM, Tupker RA (2008) Patient's estimation of efficacy of various hyperhidrosis treatments in a dermatological clinic. Acta Derm Venereol 88(4):356–362. https://doi.org/10.2340/00015555-0440

Augustin M, Radtke MA, Herberger K, Kornek T, Heigel H, Schaefer I (2013) Prevalence and disease burden of hyperhidrosis in the adult population. Dermatology 227(1):10–13. https://doi.org/10.1159/000351292

Basra MKA, Shahrukh M (2009) Burden of skin diseases. Expert Rev Pharmacoecon Outcomes Res 9(3):271–283

Bechara FG, Gambichler T, Bader A, Sand M, Altmeyer P, Hoffmann K (2007) Assessment of quality of life in patients with primary axillary hyperhidrosis before and after suction-curettage. J Am Acad Dermatol 57(2):207–212. https://doi.org/10.1016/j.jaad.2007.01.035

Beltraminelli H, Itin P (2008) Skin and psyche – from the surface to the depth of the inner world. J Dtsch Dermatol Ges 6(1):8–14. https://doi.org/10.1111/j.1610-0387.2007.06406.x

Bhatti ZU, Salek MS, Finlay AY (2011) Major life changing decisions and cumulative life course impairment. J Eur Acad Dermatol Venereol 25(2):245–246. https://doi.org/10.1111/j.1468-3083.2010.03930.x

Both H, Essink-Bot M-L, Busschbach J, Nijsten T (2007) Critical review of generic and dermatology-specific health-related quality of life instruments. J Investig Dermatol 127(12):2726–2739

Bowen GA (2006) Grounded theory and sensitizing concepts. Int J Qual Methods 5(3):12–23. https://doi.org/10.1177/160940690600500304

Bowling A (2009) Research methods in health: investigating health and health services. McGraw-Hill Education, New York. https://books.google.de/books?id=D7PlCQAAQBAJ

Braun V, Clarke V (2006) Using thematic analysis in psychology. Qual Res Psychol 3(2): 77–101

Campanati A, Penna L, Guzzo T, Menotta L, Silvestri B, Lagalla G, Gesuita R, Offidani A (2003) Quality-of-life assessment in patients with hyperhidrosis before and after treatment with botulinum toxin: results of an open-label study. Clin Ther 25(1):298–308

Campanati A, Sandroni L, Gesuita R, Giuliano A, Giuliodori K, Marconi B, Ganzetti G, Offidani A (2010) Treatment of focal idiopathic hyperhidrosis with botulinum toxin type A: clinical predictive factors of relapse-free survival. J Eur Acad Dermatol Venereol. https://doi.org/10.1111/j.1468-3083.2010.03880.x

Chren MM (2005) Measurement of vital signs for skin diseases. J Invest Dermatol 125(4):viii–viix. https://doi.org/10.1111/j.0022-202X.2005.23796.x

Cinà CS, Clase CM (1999) The illness intrusiveness rating scale: a measure of severity in individuals with hyperhidrosis. Qual Life Res 8(8):693–698. https://doi.org/10.1023/a:1008968401068

DeVellis RF (2016) Scale development: theory and applications. Applied social research methods. SAGE Publications, Thousands Oaks. https://books.google.de/books?id=48ACCwAAQBAJ

Finlay AY, Ryan TJ (1996) Disability and handicap in dermatology. Int J Dermatol 35(5): 305–311

Finlay AY (1998) Quality of life assessments in dermatology. Semin Cutan Med Surg 17: 291–296

Frost MH, Reeve BB, Liepa AM, Stauffer JW, Hays RD, Mayo/FDA Patient-Reported Outcomes Consensus Meeting Group (2007) What is sufficient evidence for the reliability and validity of patient-reported outcome measures? Value Health 10:94–105

Fujimoto T, Kawahara K, Yokozeki H (2013) Epidemiological study and considerations of primary focal hyperhidrosis in japan: from Questionnaire Analysis. J Dermatol 40(11):886–890. https://doi.org/10.1111/1346-8138.12258

Glogau RG (2001) Treatment of palmar hyperhidrosis with botulinum toxin. Semin Cutan Med Surg 20(2):101–108

Golics CJ, Basra MKA, Finlay AY, Salek MS (2009) Adolescents with skin disease have specific quality of life issues. Dermatology 218(4):357–366

Hamm H, Naumann MK, Kowalski JW, Kutt S, Kozma C, Teale C (2006) Primary focal hyperhidrosis: disease characteristics and functional impairment. Dermatology 212(4):343–353. https://doi.org/10.1159/000092285

Haynes SN, Richard D, Kubany ES (1995) Content validity in psychological assessment: a functional approach to concepts and methods. Psychol Assess 7(3):238

Hornberger J, Grimes K, Naumann M, Glaser DA, Lowe NJ, Naver H, Ahn S, Stolman LP (2004) Recognition, diagnosis, and treatment of primary focal hyperhidrosis. J Am Acad Dermatol 51(2):274–286. https://doi.org/10.1016/j.jaad.2003.12.029

Hund M, Kinkelin I, Naumann M, Hamm H (2002) Definition of axillary hyperhidrosis by gravimetric assessment. Arch Dermatol 138(4):539

Innocenzi D, Lupi F, Bruni F, Frasca M, Panetta C, Milani M (2005) Efficacy of a new aluminium salt thermophobic foam in the treatment of axillary and palmar primary hyperhidrosis: a pilot exploratory trial. Curr Med Res Opin 21(12):1949–1953. https://doi.org/10.1185/030079905x74899

Jowett S, Ryan T (1985) Skin disease and handicap: an analysis of the impact of skin conditions. Soc Sci Med 20(4):425–429. https://doi.org/10.1016/0277-9536(85)90021-8

Kalkan MT, Aydemir EH, Karakoc Y, Koerpinar MA (1998) The measurement of sweat intensity using a new technique. Turk J Med Sci 28:515–518

Kamudoni P, Mueller B, Halford J, Schouveller A, Stacey B, Salek MS (2017) The impact of hyperhidrosis on patients' daily life and quality of life: a qualitative investigation. Health Qual Life Outcomes 15(1):121. https://doi.org/10.1186/s12955-017-0693-x.

Keller S, Bello R, Vibert B, Swergold G, Burk R (2009) Diagnosis of Palmar hyperhidrosis via questionnaire without physical examination. Clin Auton Res 19(3):175–181. https://doi.org/10.1007/s10286-009-0006-5

Kim WO, Kil HK, Yoon KB, Yoo JH (2010) Treatment of generalized hyperhidrosis with oxybutynin in post-menopausal patients. Acta Derm Venereol 90(3):291–293. https://doi.org/10.2340/00015555-0828

Lima SO, Aragao JF, Machado Neto J, Almeida KB, Menezes LM, Santana VR (2015) Research of primary hyperhidrosis in students of medicine of the state of Sergipe, Brazil. An Bras Dermatol 90(5):661–665. https://doi.org/10.1590/abd1806-4841.20153859

Liu Y, Bahar R, Kalia S, Huang RY, Phillips A, Mingwan S, Yang S, Zhang X, Zhou P, Zhou Y (2016) Hyperhidrosis prevalence and demographical characteristics in dermatology outpatients in Shanghai and Vancouver. PLoS One 11(4):e0153719

Lohr KN (2002) Assessing health status and quality-of-life instruments: attributes and review criteria. Qual Life Res 11(3):193–205. https://doi.org/10.1023/a:1015291021312.

Lupin M, Hong HC, O'Shaughnessy KF (2014) Long-term efficacy and quality of life assessment for treatment of axillary hyperhidrosis with a microwave device. Dermatol Surg 40(7):805–807. https://doi.org/10.1111/dsu.0000000000000041

Muller C, Berensmeier A, Hamm H, Dirschka T, Reich K, Fischer T, Rzany B (2012) Efficacy and safety of methantheline bromide (vagantin((R))) in axillary and palmar hyperhidrosis: results from a multicenter, randomized, placebo-controlled trial. J Eur Acad Dermatol Venereol 27(10):1278–1284. https://doi.org/10.1111/j.1468-3083.2012.04708.x.

Mullin PA, Lohr KN, Bresnahan BW, McNulty P (2000) Applying cognitive design principles to formatting HRQOL instruments. Qual Life Res 9(1):13–27

Norquist JM, Girman C, Fehnel S, DeMuro-Mercon C, Santanello N (2011) Choice of recall period for patient-reported outcome (PRO) measures: criteria for consideration. Qual Life Res 10:1013–1021

Ohhashi T, Sakaguchi M, Tsuda T (1998) Human perspiration measurement. Physiol Meas 19(4):449–461

Park EJ, Han KR, Choi H, Kim do W, Kim C (2010) An epidemiological study of hyperhidrosis patients visiting the Ajou University Hospital Hyperhidrosis Center in Korea. J Korean Med Sci 25(5):772–775. https://doi.org/10.3346/jkms.2010.25.5.772

Patrick DL, Burke LB, Gwaltney CJ, Leidy NK, Martin ML, Molsen E, Ring L (2011a) Content validity – establishing and reporting the evidence in newly developed patient-reported outcomes (PRO) instruments for medical product evaluation: ISPOR PRO good research practices task force report: part 2 – assessing respondent understanding. Value Health 14(8):978–988

Patrick DL, Burke LB, Gwaltney CJ, Leidy NK, Martin ML, Molsen E, Ring L (2011b) Content validity – establishing and reporting the evidence in newly developed patient-reported outcomes (PRO) instruments for medical product evaluation: ISPOR PRO good research practices task force report: part 1 – eliciting concepts for a new PRO instrument. Value Health 14(8):967–977. https://doi.org/10.1016/j.jval.2011.06.014.

Rosell K, Kristina HMNELIUS, Swartling C (2012) Botulinum toxin type A and B improve quality of life in patients with axillary and palmar hyperhidrosis. Acta Derm Venereol 93(3):335–339

Rothman M, Burke L, Erickson P, Leidy NK, Patrick DL, Petrie CD (2009) Use of existing patient-reported outcome (PRO) instruments and their modification: the ISPOR good research practices for evaluating and documenting content validity for the use of existing instruments and their modification PRO task force report. Value Health 12(8):1075–1083

Rothman ML, Beltran P, Cappelleri JC, Lipscomb J, Teschendorf B, F. D. A. Patient-Reported Outcomes Consensus Meeting Group the Mayo (2007) Patient-reported outcomes: conceptual issues. Value Health 10:S66–S75. https://doi.org/10.1111/j.1524-4733.2007.00269.x

Ruchinskas R (2007) Hyperhidrosis and anxiety: chicken or egg? Dermatology 214(3):195–196. https://doi.org/10.1159/000099581

Solish N (2006) Assessing hyperhidrosis disease severity and impact on quality of life. Cutis 77(Suppl. 5):17–27

Solish N, Benohanian A, Kowalski JW (2005) Prospective open-label study of botulinum toxin type A in patients with axillary hyperhidrosis: effects on functional impairment and quality of life. Dermatol Surg 31(4):405–413

Streiner DL, Norman GR (2008) Health measurement scales: a practical guide to their development and use. Oxford University Press, Oxford. http://books.google.co.uk/books?id=UbKijeRqndwC

Strutton DR, Kowalski JW, Glaser DA, Stang PE (2004) US Prevalence of hyperhidrosis and impact on individuals with axillary hyperhidrosis: results from a national survey. J Am Acad Dermatol 51(2):241–248. https://doi.org/10.1016/j.jaad.2003.12.040

Swartling C, Naver H, Lindberg M (2001) Botulinum A toxin improves life quality in severe primary focal hyperhidrosis. Eur J Neurol 8(3):247–252

Tan SR, Solish N (2002) Long-term efficacy and quality of life in the treatment of focal hyperhidrosis with botulinum toxin A. Dermatol Surg 28(6):495–499

Thomas M, Pieretti L, Swaile D, Capretta A, Hill T (2006) Panel discussions among hyperhidrosis patients to assess lifestyle limitations, treatment regimes, and compensating behaviors, 64th annual meeting of the American Academy of Dermatology, 3–7 Mar, 2006, San Fransisco

Content Validation by Patients and Experts: Is the PRO Measure Fit for Purpose?

4

The standardised measurement of most PRO concepts is based on a presumption that the content of the instruments (or questionnaires) used is a good indicator of the underlying unobservable target concept (Wynd et al. 2003). In addition to other types of data, this assumption needs to be supported by evidence of content validity, i.e. the 'complete relevance' of the content to the target population and how adequately it represents the underlying construct. Without such evidence, the definition of the underlying concept being measured becomes ambiguous, and the scores would be rendered meaningless (Haynes et al. 1995). While evidence ensuring content validity is generated through inclusion of input from patients in defining the content of the measure, confirming that 'complete relevance' has been attained is crucial. This is addressed in Steps 5 and 6 of the roadmap, where respondent understanding of the measure and comprehensives is explicitly explored in Step 5, with practicality and acceptability explored in Step 6. Importantly, both steps allow the PRO measure to be fine-tuned to address any issues uncovered in the steps. These steps are illustrated in the current chapter, based on the patient and clinician panels conducted to assess the content validity of the HidroQoL as well as a pilot test of the measure assessing the practicality and acceptability of the HidroQoL.

Step 5: Refining the Content of the PRO Measure

Formally, content validity of an instrument reflects the extent to which it represents the most relevant and important aspects of a concept in the context of a given measurement application (Magasi et al. 2011). Ensuring content validity, therefore, requires that the content domain is adequately sampled suggesting a rigorous instrument development process (Nunnally and Bernstein 1994).

Similar to other psychometric properties, content validity is specific to particular measurement aims, usage, construct being assessed and target population, hence the need for clearly articulating these (Terwee et al. 2007). In particular, experts judge the appropriateness and relevance of the content in relation to the construct being

P. Kamudoni et al., *Living with Chronic Disease: Measuring Important Patient-Reported Outcomes*, https://doi.org/10.1007/978-981-10-8414-0_4

measured and the considerations listed above (Streiner and Norman 2008). This process, then, is the first 'proof of concept' that the instrument's content is connected to the construct being measured. Without such evidence, construct validity and the meaning attached to the instrument's scores (interpretability) may not be established (Haynes et al. 1995). On the other hand, an instrument demonstrating content validity is more likely to reflect strong construct validity, interpretability besides superior acceptability and practicality as it would tap into the most relevant issues for both the construct and patients, also rendering the measure more interesting to patients.

The scope of an instrument's content considered during content validation studies should extend beyond just items and their responses. All elements of the instrument that would influence the data collected should be included (Haynes et al. 1995). Responses and collected data may be influenced, for example, by the structure of the instrument (i.e. the instructions, response formats, and frame of references) and technical quality of the measure, apart from the relevance of the content to a given patient population (Patrick et al. 2011).

Case Study: Evaluating the Content of the HidroQoL

This study examined whether the HidroQoL adequately addressed important aspects of QoL relevant to hyperhidrosis patients and whether all other aspects of the instrument such as content's structure and technical quality supported this. Content validity was formally assessed by expert panels to ensure relevance of the content, specifically focusing on (1) whether the content was relevant to patients with hyperhidrosis and the conceptual understanding of QoL in hyperhidrosis; (2) the adequacy with which the new instrument represented the concept of hyperhidrosis quality of life, i.e. whether some aspects were not covered; and (3) the appropriateness of the layout, recall period and technical quality of the new instrument for assessing hyperhidrosis-QoL.

Each item was evaluated on multiple criteria:

- *Language clarity*—The sentence and wording of each item should be clear, understandable, straightforward and simple. Phrases and wording should be unambiguous and jargon free and should be understood by someone with a reading ability of a 12-year old (Streiner and Norman 2008).
- *Completeness*—The sentences should be complete and not broken and should end appropriately, comprehensively addressing the idea they are covering (Guyatt et al. 1993).
- *Relevance*—Each item should reflect an aspect of HRQoL of importance to the target patient population, thus also relevant to the construct being measured (Leidy et al. 1999).
- *Scaling*—This represents how the actual responses of the patients will be measured. The choice of the response format, number and labelling of response categories must fit the items and be appropriate to the construct being measured (DeVellis 2016).

In addition, various aspects of the content were considered for appropriateness:

- *Layout of questionnaire*—the graphical structure and design must lend themselves to a natural flow through the questionnaire (Mullin et al. 2000) including pagination, font size and font styles.
- *Instructions*—provide important orientation to the patient regarding what is being measured, the frame of reference to apply when providing responses and how to choose between response categories (Patrick et al. 2011). These need to be adequate, clear and appropriately located.
- *Frame of reference or recall period*—this defines the period of time patients need to refer to when providing their responses, i.e. the recall period (Norquist et al. 2011). It has to be suitable for the construct being measured (HRQoL impact), the characteristics of the disease, the treatment and duration of treatment effect, the intended number of assessments and the target population (Norquist et al. 2011).

Methods

Part I: Performing Expert Panels for Content Validation

Five dermatologists from leading centres were invited to participate in the content validation of the HidroQoL. Each panel member was provided a copy of the developmental HidroQoL and the content validation questionnaire. The content validation questionnaire evaluated each of the 47 items of the HidroQoL on 4 aspects, language clarity, completeness, relevance and scaling, as previously defined. Each of these aspects was rated on a 4-point Likert scale as 1 = strongly disagree, 2 = disagree, 3 = agree and 4 = strongly agree, for all items. Additional space was provided for open-ended feedback or suggestions for each item as well as the entire questionnaire. A session was conducted in the form of a panel discussion to assess the adequacy of all aspects of the HidroQoL as done by the specialist panel. Panel sessions were tape recorded and later transcribed. Transcripts were analysed for the major issues and decisions relating to each aspect of content assessed.

Part II: Working with Patients During Content Validation

In this novel approach, patient engagement was initiated and a patient-expert panel was developed. Similar to the specialist expert panel, an invitation was made to seven patients who had lived with the condition for at least 10 years and who were English native speakers, through the International Hyperhidrosis Society (IHHS). A minimum of three patients should be accepted for such panels, although having five or more reduces chance agreement (Lynn 1986).

A session was conducted in the form of a panel discussion to assess the adequacy of all aspects of the HidroQoL as done in specialist panel. In order to assess whether the construct of hyperhidrosis-QoL was adequately covered by the developmental instrument, the panel was asked whether there were any gaps in the content or whether they would make any additions to the items. They considered the HidroQoL to cover all important HRQoL issues for patients with hyperhidrosis; thus they suggested no additions.

Part III: A Review Panel

To take into account of both specialist and patient panels, a review panel was developed. Three experts in outcomes research were invited to participate in the review process following content validation. This included a professor in health outcome measurement and two clinical researchers with experience in hyperhidrosis, one with a medical degree and the other with a pharmacy degree.

Findings

Part I: Expert Panels

Qualitative Feedback

The dermatologists' panel found the general layout of the instrument including the font style, font size and organisation of the instrument to be appropriate and adequate. The instruction *If a statement does not apply to you please mark 'not relevant'* on the first/cover page of the draft HidroQoL was considered inappropriately placed. Concerns were raised that patients might also apply this instruction to the demographics question following immediately after on the same page, resulting in confusion or mistakes in the completion of the demographic questions. The panel's recommendation was to remove this instruction from the first page but to retain it on the rest of the pages. It was suggested that the instructions on the rest of the pages of the instrument be enclosed in a border. An additional change was suggested to the instruction *The statements in this questionnaire relate to how* ***your*** *life is being affected by your excessive sweating condition (hyperhidrosis) at the moment.* Instead of emphasising the words 'your' only, the emphasis was to be placed on the entire clause *your life is being affected by your excessive sweating*.

The recall period *at the moment* was considered to be too short and impractical. It was argued that when patients are asked about how they feel at the moment, they relate to events of the preceding days. They further stated that if the instrument were to be used for monitoring of response to treatments, a day may not be long enough to observe any meaningful changes. A recall period of 1–2 weeks was suggested instead. Several issues were raised regarding the response scaling: for the general impact question, *in general, how would you rate the effect of excessive sweating on your life*, with response options (*no effect at all*, *slight*, *moderate*, *quite a bit* and *extreme*), the panel considered these to not appropriately reflect equal interval of increasing intensity. They suggested changing 'slight' to 'mild', 'quite a bit' to 'strong' and 'extreme' to 'very strong'. Furthermore, in relation to the response scaling used for the individual items, *no, not at all, a little, somewhat, quite a bit, very much* and *not applicable*, the panel made a number of points. They considered *a little* and *somewhat* to lack a clear demarcation; *quite a bit* was seen as not reflecting midway between *somewhat* and *very much*. A strong case was made against including *not relevant*.

The panel raised concerns about ambiguity between the option *no, no at all* and *not relevant*. An example given was of the item *my hobbies are affected*. Although the expectation is that only those without hobbies would choose the *not relevant* option while those with hobbies but not affected choosing *no, not at all*, respondents may easily confuse the two.

Ratings by Experts

The panel also assessed language clarity, completeness, relevance and scaling of each of the 47 individual items using a 4-point Likert scale. Mean language clarity rating was below 3 in five items including *I feel uncomfortable physically expressing affection* (mean = 2.25), *I find it difficult to cope with my condition* (2.5) and *I feel more self-conscious* (2.25). SD for 16 items exceeded the minimum threshold (SD > 0.75), including *I feel my skin is hot all the time* (SD = 1.5), *my career decisions are affected* (1.15) and *my summer activities are affected* (1.15) reflecting disagreement in the ratings. Mean relevance rating was below 3 for 16 items. The same items also had a mean language clarity or completeness rating below 3. SD of relevance rating for 20 items was above the threshold, including my choice of footwear (SD 0 1.5), *my hobbies are affected* (SD = 1.15), this also included all items showing mean score exceeding 3. All items had mean scaling rating of 3 or 4, and there were no disagreements on any item. Further, ratings were analysed using content validity index. Sixteen items had I-CVI below 1 for language clarity, including *I feel more self-conscious* (CVI = 0.25), *I find it difficult to cope with my condition* (0.25) and *I feel uncomfortable physically expressing affection* (0.25). For completeness, 12 items were below the threshold (CVI = > 1), and eight of these had also been identified with language clarity problems. Twenty items did not achieve content validity for relevance, 15 of which had shown problems for language clarity and completeness.

The items with optimal language clarity and completeness but lacking in relevance including *my choice of footwear is affected, I have difficulties with physical contact with others* and *I worry about the addition demands on my finances* were endorsed for language clarity and completeness. Only one item *I feel my skin is hot all the time* had I-CVI less than 1 for scaling.

Content validity indices were also estimated at the scale level (S-CVI/UA), for language clarity, completeness, relevance and scaling. S-CVI/UA for language clarity (66%) and completeness (74%) was below minimum threshold, while relevance and scaling aspects were above the content validity threshold. Inter-rater agreement was moderate for completeness ($r = 0.5$) and poor for relevance ($r = 0.2$) (Appendix, Table 4.2). This hints to a number of challenges associated with ascertaining the relevance quality of life issues based merely based on observation as opposed to first-hand experience from patients.

Suggestions for Improving Items

A rich set of comments were provided by the panel on 29 items. Suggestions were made to delete five items including *I feel my skin is hot all the time, I feel that I need more time for hygiene chores, I find it difficult to cope with my condition and My summer activities are affected.* In the case of the item *I find it difficult to cope with my condition,* it was argued that although the concept of coping is closely related to QoL, it relates to a different construct. The panel feared that the item *My summer activities are affected* would not reflect much sensitivity to change in clinical settings. A similar comment was made with regard to *My holidays are affected.* The item *I have problems with speaking with groups of people* was also thought to cause ambiguities in the sense that it was unclear what sort of group, whether it was the 'group factor' or the 'speaking'. More general comments were also made in relation to the level at which quality of life was being measured. Whether the PRO measure would be specific to sites/types of hyperhidrosis (e.g. axillar, palmar-plantar) or whether the measure would address HRQoL issues relevant or common to all hyperhidrosis sites/types. The choice would have implications for the content, crafting of the items, structure of the measure and ultimately, its practicality. For example, if the instrument will aim to measure hyperhidrosis-QoL at a high level, then all items must be of relevance for all forms of hyperhidrosis. Paying no attention to this intricate decision risks development of a measure that would be biased against patients with one type of hyperhidrosis over another. The panel recommended assessing hyperhidrosis at a higher level where all items would apply to all forms of hyperhidrosis.

A consideration of the overall representativeness of the HidroQoL for quality of life in hyperhidrosis was also made by the panel. The panel identified various areas as being under-represented in the content: (1) concerns related to bad odour, (2) the burden related to extra effort involved in managing hyperhidrosis (e.g. carrying second bags, towel, air conditioning, washing clothes, treatment, personal hygiene) and (3) physical discomfort associated with hyperhidrosis (e.g. being wet, cracked skin, dampness, hot). Although these issues were not included in the 47-item version of the instrument, they were, nonetheless, mentioned during qualitative study.

Part II: Patient Panels

Ratings by Patients

All 47 items had mean scores of at least three for language clarity, completeness, relevance and scaling (Appendix, Table 4.1). According to the Average Mean Deviation Index, item-level disagreement in the ratings was noted. The SD for language clarity ratings in 16 items exceeded 0.75 including for *I worry about being in places close to other people* (SD = 1.41), *I feel that I need more time for hygiene* (1.1) and *I have problems speaking with groups of people* (1.1). Similarly, SD for completeness ratings for *I feel more self-conscious* (1.34), *I worry about people's reactions* (1.34) and *I worry being in places close to other people* (1.1) and an additional 16 items were above threshold. Ratings for relevance and scaling had high SD in eight and two items, respectively. Six items had language clarity I-CVI below 0.8, including *my holiday is affected* (I-CVI = 0.6), *I have problems speaking with groups of people* (I-CVI = 0.6), *I worry being in places close to other people* and *I slide in and out of my shoes* (I-CVI = 0.6). I-CVI was below 0.8 for three items for completeness including *my holiday is affected, I worry being in places close to other people* and *I slide in and out of my shoes*, while only one item (*my eating habits are affected*) had relevance I-CVI below threshold. All items were endorsed for scaling. At the scale level, all aspects (language clarity, completeness, relevance and completeness) achieved content validity (S-CVI = 87–100%). Agreement on ratings at the scale level was also strong on all the four aspects assessed, with the coefficient of agreement ranging from 0.7 to 1 (Appendix, Table 4.2).

Suggestions for Improving Items

In addition to the individual item ratings, the experts also provided comments and suggestions pertaining to specific items as well as the whole questionnaire. Comments were given on 34 items. For example, respondents commented that they were not sure whether the item 'My holiday is affected' was asking about the actual holidays or its planning. One expert thought the item 'my self-esteem is affected' duplicates 'my self-confidence is affected'. In reference to the item 'I feel my skin is hot all the time', one panel member commented that sweating would still occur even when they felt cold. Another comment made in relation to the same item was that it was not that the skin was necessarily hot, but rather damp/wet.

Part III: Review Panel

Integrating the Results

The data collected during the content validation panels provided a wealth of information on the HidroQoL covering all aspects of the HidroQoL, for instance, recommendations related to the 'frame of reference', 'instructions', suggested items to be added and the ratings of the items of the HidroQoL. The review panel examined this data and made decisions based on the developmental goals of the HidroQoL. There was consensus to maintain the instrument's structure, the graphical design, font style and font size and presentation of the items, as originally intentioned, and moreover no changes had been suggested by the expert panels. The review panel agreed to maintain the second instruction on the front page considering its relevance to the organisation of the entire instrument, with the argument that instructions on the first page relate to the entire instrument. Instructions were maintained on every page and were placed in borders. The recommendation maintained to not specify recall period or to use 'at peak' as it was considered not to reflect the intended use of the instrument for the assessment of impact on quality of life in routine clinical practice or for research. This included the assessment of change over time or making comparisons across patients. The review panel considered two other alternatives, 'in recent times', which was considered as lacking the necessary precision and containing some ambiguity, and 'over the last two weeks' which was thought to be too long. There were strong arguments for maintaining the initial proposal of 'at the moment', including the precision in assessing the patient's condition at the time of measurement. An additional consideration was the nature of the impacts of hyperhidrosis which may be felt on a longer time horizon. Rather than 'at the moment', the review panel therefore agreed on 'in the last 7 days including today' as the frame of reference.

Additionally, as recommended by the dermatologist panel, the 'not relevant' response category was removed to minimise the risk of satisficing and measurement errors. In order to address the ambiguities surrounding the demarcation between 'Quite a bit' and 'very much' as pointed out by the experts, further consultations were made. Two experts on patient-reported outcome instrument development were consulted on whether the response options were clear and represented equal intervals of increasing intensity. They considered the response categorisation to be appropriate and reflecting widely used response categorisation. On this basis, the review panel maintained the response categorisation.

The review panel agreed to delete one item *I find it difficult to cope with my condition*, given the possibility that it might be tapping into a related yet different construct than quality of life (Appendix, Table 4.3). Three new items were added (1) *I worry about my body odour*, (2) *I worry about my condition in the future* and (3) *I worry about people's reaction* to improve coverage of the hyperhidrosis quality of life. A further 17 items were revised, for instance, the item *my holidays are affected* was changed to *my holidays are affected (e.g. planning, activities)*; *I have problems speaking with groups of people* was amended to *I avoid public speaking (e.g. doing presentations)*. With a developmental goal that the HidroQoL would be relevant for patients with hyperhidrosis of all forms (e.g. palmar, feet, axillary, facial) and with considerations of practicality and applicability, it was decided that the measure will assess hyperhidrosis-QoL at a higher hierarchical level, with the implication that (1) the items included would need to have relevance for all hyperhidrosis forms and (2) the actual crafting of the items would have to reflect the same. Revisions to the HidroQoL items following the content validation panel are reported in Appendix, Table 4.3.

Naming the New PRO Instrument

Deciding on the name for the new instrument took a number of factors into consideration: (1) to be capable of hinting on the underlying concept being measured by the instrument, (2) the way that the construct was going to be measured and (3) ultimately to be easy to remember. It was agreed to include 'quality of life' in the name to reflect that the measure purports to measure this construct.

It was agreed further to include 'hyperhidrosis' in the name to emphasise the focus of the instrument, i.e. disease-specific quality of life of hyperhidrosis patients. Finally, the team debated on whether to use profile or index as a suffix. The suffix Index was chosen to reflect the intended measurement model, to hint on the availability of a single score that sums up the patients quality of life. Therefore, the full title chosen for the new instrument was 'Hyperhidrosis Quality of Life Index'. The acronym HidroQoL was chosen as a combination of 'Hidro' reflecting water and 'QoL' reflecting quality of life. It was thought that this would also be easy to remember as a measure of HRQoL in hyperhidrosis. Following thorough consideration of the findings from the expert panels, the revisions decided by the review panel led to the developmental version of the new instrument, the HidroQoL. This included 49 items scored on a common 5-point Likert scale. Field testing and further validation studies carried out later used this version.

Step 6: Explore practicality and applicability

Among other attributes, user-friendliness and suitability of a PRO to a specific use setting of use represents an important aspect which must be deliberately considered in the measure development process. For instance, measures developed for use in routine clinical practice must demonstrate feasibility in that setting considering time constraints as well as relatively lower skill levels in data management (Higginson and Carr 2001). While practicality and applicability are somewhat addressed through the content validation panel, pretesting of a new instrument in a small sample (~15–20 respondents) may serve a useful purpose for troubleshooting of these aspects in the target population.

Case Study: Pretesting of the HidroQoL

It is expected that the HidroQoL would be practical and applicable to be used in the population.

Prior to larger studies to test psychometric attributes, an electronic/web version of HidroQoL pretested with 20 patients who were members of the IHHS. In addition to completion of the HidroQoL, the participants also provided their views on the practicality and applicability of the measure using a bespoke feedback questionnaire (see Appendix—Box 4.1—for sample pretesting questions). In addition, the usability of the electronic measure was also tested.

Overall, 95% of respondents ($n = 19$) considered the new measure to be relevant, easy to understand and easy to complete, while 90% ($n = 18$) agreed that the measure had appropriate length and was relevant. The average completion time for the measure (i.e. developmental version of the measure with 49 items) was 5 ± 4 min.

Ninety-five percent ($n = 19$) of the participants found the website to be easy to use, while 80% found it easy to navigate through. The layout of the instructions, responses and questions was considered appropriate by 90% of the participants. Free comments provided by the patients suggested that there were no major issues related to the design or content of the measure:

- 'Thanks a lot'.
- 'Some of the questions do not apply to as I sweat mostly from the head'.
- 'Not a bad survey. One or two vague questions such as "do I feel hopeless"…do I interpret that to mean life? Also one of the biggest negatives with my palmar hyperhidrosis is skin peeling/blistering but the only question that referenced skin condition I think was "is your skin uncomfortable" or something to that effect. Also no question on how you are coping with hyperhidrosis'.

Subsequently, results from the pilot testing were reviewed by the research team to consider any necessary revisions. No revisions were deemed necessary. For instance, a number of items related to dealing with hyperhidrosis such as 'I worry about the additional activities in dealing with my condition' were considered adequate for capturing aspects of disease burden associated with living with the condition. Issues directly related to skin symptoms or coping were considered to be out of scope for the measure.

Concluding Remarks

A formal statistical test for assessing the content validity of a PRO measure does not exist. The involvement of patients in concept elicitation provides supportive evidence of content validity. More formally content validity may be assessed by content experts (Streiner and Norman 2008)—who may be therapeutic area experts or patients—who rate the content on specified criteria.

This chapter has presented an illustration of how the content validity of a PRO measure may be assessed using expert panels, using work done in the development of the HidroQoL as an example. In our example, various attributes of an instrument including the layout, the instructions, frame of reference, response scaling as well as the individual items were evaluated systematically by two expert panels. Recommendations by the expert panels were then used by the review panel to revise the HidroQoL measure.

Overall, the HidroQoL met content validity criteria for language clarity, completeness, relevance and scaling based on the judgement of the patient panel. Relevance and scaling were also endorsed in the dermatologist panel, while language clarity and completeness were not supported by this panel. As a result, one item was deleted, twenty-nine were revised, and three were added, resulting in a 49-item developmental instrument, scored on a 5-point Likert scale.

The two panels considered the formatting and design of the HidroQoL appropriate, allowing a natural flow through the questionnaire. On recommendation of the panels, various changes were made, for example, instructions were revised changing the emphasis on particular phrases and including instructions on each page throughout the instrument. The proposed frame of reference, 'at the moment', was thought to be too short and not consistent with the nature of the impact of hyperhidrosis or its treatment by the patient panel. The patients suggested not including any defined recall period. Clinician experts suggested a 1-week recall, on the basis that patients tend to think about the recent past even when asked about today. The frame of reference was therefore defined revised to 'in the last seven days including today'.

The involvement of patients as experts at this stage in the PRO measure development is important. Apart from their unique expertise, their first-hand experience of living with a condition, their input is key to ensure patient friendliness and practicality. In our example, the two panels rated relevance differently; the patient's panel endorsed all items except 'my holiday is affected', while the dermatologists endorsed only 27 out of the 49 items. Differences in how medical practitioners and patients with skin disease evaluate their own quality of life have been observed before (Jemec and Wulf 1996). Not all patient experiences may be observable to the clinician.

Discussion among experts during the panels contributed insights and ideas to content development of the HidroQoL; focused discussions tend to generate rich and unique data as discussion members contribute and respond to each other's comments (Krueger 1994). This suggests that allowing discussion among experts in addition to a quantitative assessment using a questionnaire may be of great value.

Appendix

Content verification of the 47-item prototype HidroQoL by patients and Experts

Table 4.1 Patient panel ratings of language clarity, completeness, relevance and scaling of the HidroQoL

		Language		Completeness		Relevance		Scaling		I-CVI			
	Instrument item	Mean	SD	Mean	SD	Mean	SD	Mean	SD	Lan	Com	Rel	Scal
1	My choice of clothing is affected	4	0	4	0	4	0	4	0	1	1	1	1
2	My choice of footwear is affected	4	0	4	0	4	0	4	0	1	1	1	1
3	My holiday is affected	3.2	1.1	3.2	1.1	3.8	0.45	4	0	0.6	0.6	1	1
4	I have difficulties gripping objects	3.6	0.89	3.6	0.89	4	0	4	0	0.8	0.8	1	1
5	I have difficulties handling money	4	0	4	0	4	0	4	0	1	1	1	1
6	I have difficulties with physical contact with others	3.6	0.89	4	0	4	0	4	0	0.8	1	1	1
7	My hobbies are affected	3.8	0.45	4	0	4	0	4	0	1	1	1	1
8	I have problems speaking with groups of people	3.2	1.1	3.6	0.89	3.6	0.89	4	0	0.6	0.8	0.8	1
9	My physical activities are affected	3.8	0.45	4	0	4	0	4	0	1	1	1	1
10	My outdoor activities are affected	3.8	0.45	4	0	4	0	4	0	1	1	1	1
11	My everyday housework is affected	4	0	4	0	4	0	4	0	1	1	1	1
12	I find it hard to handle paper	4	0	4	0	4	0	4	0	1	1	1	1
13	My career decisions are affected	3.6	0.89	4	0	4	0	4	0	0.8	1	1	1
14	My work is affected	3.6	0.89	4	0	4	0	4	0	0.8	1	1	1
15	I have difficulties with using touch technologies	4	0	4	0	4	0	4	0	1	1	1	1
16	My relationships with others are affected	3.6	0.89	4	0	4	0	4	0	0.8	1	1	1
17	I feel embarrassed	3.6	0.89	4	0	4	0	3.6	0.89	0.8	1	1	0.8
18	I do not socialise as much as I would like to	4	0	4	0	4	0	4	0	1	1	1	1
19	I avoid meeting people	4	0	4	0	4	0	4	0	1	1	1	1
20	I avoid going out	4	0	4	0	4	0	4	0	1	1	1	1
21	I feel nervous	4	0	3.6	0.89	3.6	0.89	4	0	1	0.8	0.8	1

(continued)

Table 4.1 (continued)

	Instrument item	Language		Completeness		Relevance		Scaling		I-CVI			
		Mean	SD	Mean	SD	Mean	SD	Mean	SD	Lan	Com	Rel	Scal
22	I feel hopeless	4	0	3.6	0.89	3.6	0.89	4	0	1	0.8	0.8	1
23	I feel sad	4	0	3.6	0.89	3.6	0.89	4	0	1	0.8	0.8	1
24	I feel depressed	4	0	3.6	0.89	3.6	0.89	4	0	1	0.8	0.8	1
25	I feel frustrated	4	0	3.6	0.89	3.6	0.89	4	0	1	0.8	0.8	1
26	My confidence is affected	4	0	4	0	4	0	4	0	1	1	1	1
27	My self-esteem is affected	4	0	4	0	4	0	4	0	1	1	1	1
28	My whole life is affected	4	0	4	0	4	0	4	0	1	1	1	1
29	Sweating is constantly on my mind	4	0	4	0	4	0	4	0	1	1	1	1
30	I avoid taking on new challenges	3.8	0.45	4	0	4	0	4	0	1	1	1	1
31	My summer activities are affected	3.6	0.89	4	0	4	0	4	0	0.8	1	1	1
32	I feel more self-conscious	3.8	0.45	3.4	1.34	4	0	4	0	1	0.8	1	1
33	My appearance is affected	3.8	0.45	3.6	0.89	4	0	4	0	1	0.8	1	1
34	I feel uncomfortable physically expressing affection	3.4	0.89	3.6	0.89	4	0	4	0	0.8	0.8	1	1
35	I worry about people's reactions	3.8	0.45	3.4	1.34	4	0	4	0	1	0.8	1	1
36	My sex life is affected	4	0	4	0	4	0	4	0	1	1	1	1
37	I worry about leaving sweat marks in public places	4	0	4	0	4	0	4	0	1	1	1	1
38	I worry being in places close to other people	3	1.41	3.2	1.1	4	0	4	0	0.6	0.6	1	1
39	My eating habits are affected	3.2	1.1	3.4	0.89	3.2	1.1	4	0	0.6	0.8	0.6	1
40	I slide in and out of my shoes	3	1	3.2	1.1	3.6	0.89	3.6	0.89	0.6	0.6	0.8	0.8
41	I have problems with being barefoot	3.8	0.45	3.8	0.45	4	0	4	0	1	1	1	1
42	My eyes get irritated	3.4	0.89	3.4	0.89	3.8	0.45	4	0	0.8	0.8	1	1
43	I feel my skin is hot all the time	3.4	0.89	3.6	0.89	3.6	0.55	4	0	0.8	0.8	1	1
44	I worry about the extra demands on my finances	3.8	0.45	3.6	0.89	4	0	4	0	1	0.8	1	1
45	I find it difficult to cope with my condition	4	0	4	0	4	0	4	0	1	1	1	1
46	I find it difficult to do things without planning in advance	3.8	0.45	4	0	4	0	4	0	1	1	1	1
47	I feel that I need more time for hygiene chores	3.2	1.1	3.4	0.89	4	0	4	0	0.6	0.8	1	1

Note: Lan, language clarity; Com, completeness; Rel, relevance; Scal, scaling

Table 4.2 (a) Level of agreement and content validity index for the panel of patients and (b) level of agreement and content validity index for the panel of dermatologists

	CVI[a], %	AC1, r^b
Language clarity	87	0.7
Completeness	94	0.8
Relevance	98	0.9
Scaling	100	1
Language clarity	66	0.5
Completeness	74	0.6
Relevance	89	0.2
Scaling	98	1

[a]Content Validity Index
[b]Gwet's AC1 coefficient of agreement

Table 4.3 Revision to the items of the HidroQoL following content validation panels

	Before content validation	After content validation
1	My choice of clothing is affected	My choice of clothing is affected
2	My choice of footwear is affected	My choice of footwear is affected
3	My holiday is affected	My holidays are affected (e.g. planning, activities)
4	I have difficulties gripping objects	I have difficulties holding objects
5	I have difficulties handling money	I have difficulties handling money
6	I have difficulties with physical contact with others	I find it hard to touch other people
7	My hobbies are affected	My hobbies are affected
8	I have problems speaking with groups of people	I avoid public speaking (e.g. during presentations)
9	My physical activities are affected	My physical activities are affected
10	My outdoor activities are affected	My outdoor activities are affected
11	My everyday housework is affected	My everyday housework is affected
12	I find it hard to handle paper	I find it hard to handle paper
13	My career decisions are affected	My career decisions are affected (e.g. career choice)
14	My work is affected	My work is affected
15	I have difficulties with using touch technologies	I have difficulties using touch technologies (e.g. computer keyboard, smart phones)
16	My relationships with others are affected	My personal relationships are affected
17	I feel embarrassed	I feel embarrassed
18	I do not socialise as much as I would like to	I do not socialise as much as I would like to
19	I avoid meeting people	I avoid meeting new people

(continued)

Table 4.3 (continued)

	Before content validation	After content validation
20	I avoid going out	I avoid going out
21	I feel nervous	I feel nervous
22	I feel hopeless	I feel hopeless
23	I feel sad	I feel sad
24	I feel depressed	I feel depressed
25	I feel frustrated	I feel frustrated
26	My confidence is affected	My self-confidence is affected
27	My self-esteem is affected	My self-esteem is affected
28	My whole life is affected	My whole life is affected
29	Sweating is constantly on my mind	Sweating is constantly on my mind
30	I avoid taking on new challenges	I avoid taking on new challenges
31	My summer activities are affected	My summer activities are affected
32	I feel more self-conscious	I feel self-conscious
33	My appearance is affected	My appearance is affected
34	I feel uncomfortable physically expressing affection	I feel uncomfortable physically expressing affection (e.g. hugging and cuddling)
35	I worry about people's reactions	I worry about people's reactions
36	My sex life is affected	My sex life is affected
37	I worry about leaving sweat marks in public places	I worry about leaving sweating marks on things
38	I worry being in places close to other people	I find it hard to be near other people
39	My eating habits are affected	My choice of food and drinks is affected
40	I slide in and out of my shoes	I feel uncomfortable in my shoes
41	I have problems with being barefoot	I have problems with being barefooted
42	My eyes get irritated	My eyes feel irritated
43	I feel my skin is hot all the time	My skin feels uncomfortable
44	I worry about the extra demands on my finances	I worry about the additional money spent in dealing with my condition
45	I find it difficult to cope with my condition	[item deleted]
46	I find it difficult to do things without planning in advance	I find it hard to do things without planning in advance
47	I feel that I need more time for hygiene chores	I worry about the additional time spend in dealing with my condition
		I worry about my body odour
		I worry about my condition in the future
		I worry about the additional chores in dealing with my condition

Practicality Questions

Box 4.1 Sample Questions Used in Pretesting of New PRO Questionnaires: Presented for the Overall Questionnaire or the Individual Items

1. Did you experience any difficulties in understanding the instructions? [*If yes, which specific words or elements were difficult?*]
2. Did you experience any difficulties in understanding or completing the items in this questionnaire? [*If yes, which specific items, and what difficulties did you encounter?*]
3. What are your views regarding the number of items in this questionnaire?
4. Are there any important aspects (items) currently not covered in the questionnaire, which should be added to the questionnaire?
5. Are there any items currently in the questionnaire, which are not relevant and should be removed?

References

DeVellis RF (2016) Scale development: theory and applications. Applied social research methods. SAGE Publications, London. https://books.google.de/books?id=48ACCwAAQBAJ

Guyatt GH, Feeny DH, Patrick DL (1993) Measuring health-related quality of life. Ann Intern Med 118(8):622–629

Haynes SN, Richard D, Kubany ES (1995) Content validity in psychological assessment: a functional approach to concepts and methods. Psychol Assess 7(3):238

Higginson IJ, Carr AJ (2001) Measuring quality of life: using quality of life measures in the clinical setting. BMJ 322(7297):1297

Jemec GBE, Wulf HC (1996) Patient–physician consensus on quality of life in dermatology. Clin Exp Dermatol 21(3):177–179

Krueger RA (1994) Focus groups: practical guide for applied research. Sage Publications Ltd., London. http://books.google.de/books?id=ak9UcAAACAAJ

Leidy NK, Revicki DA, Genesté B (1999) Recommendations for evaluating the validity of quality of life claims for labeling and promotion. Value Health 2(2):113–127

Lynn MR (1986) Determination and quantification of content validity. Nurs Res 35(6):382–385

Magasi S, Ryan G, Revicki D, Lenderking W, Hays RD, Brod M, Snyder C, Boers M, Cella D (2011) Content validity of patient-reported outcome measures: perspectives from a PROMIS meeting. Qual Life Res 21:739–746

Mullin PA, Lohr KN, Bresnahan BW, McNulty P (2000) Applying cognitive design principles to formatting HRQOL instruments. Qual Life Res 9(1):13–27

Norquist JM, Girman C, Fehnel S, DeMuro-Mercon C, Santanello N (2011) Choice of recall period for patient-reported outcome (PRO) measures: criteria for consideration. Qual Life Res 21:1013–1020

Nunnally JC, Bernstein IH (1994) Psychometric theory. McGraw-Hill, London. http://books.google.de/books?id=r0fuAAAAMAAJ

Patrick DL, Burke LB, Gwaltney CJ, Leidy NK, Martin ML, Molsen E, Ring L (2011) Content validity – establishing and reporting the evidence in newly developed patient-reported outcomes (PRO) instruments for medical product evaluation: ISPOR PRO good research practices task force report: part 2 – assessing respondent understanding. Value Health 14(8):978–988

Streiner DL, Norman GR (2008) Health measurement scales: a practical guide to their development and use. Oxford University Press, Oxford. http://books.google.co.uk/books?id=UbKijeRqndwC

Terwee CB, Bot SDM, De Boer MR, van der Windt DAWM, Knol DL, Dekker J, Bouter LM, De Vet HCW (2007) Quality criteria were proposed for measurement properties of health status questionnaires. J Clin Epidemiol 60(1):34–42

Wynd CA, Schmidt B, Schaefer MA (2003) Two quantitative approaches for estimating content validity. West J Nurs Res 25(5):508–518

Applying Modern Test Theory in PRO Measure Development: Rasch Modelling

5

This chapter is intended to describe how approaches based on Item Response Theory (IRT) may be applied to PRO measure development and represents Step 7 of the PRO roadmap – instrument fine-tuning and assessment of item performance. A practical example based on item-level analysis and Rasch model analyses performed on the HidroQoL is presented in the first section of the chapter, Part I. The type of questions that such methods may help to address and the techniques in undertaking IRT analyses are illustrated. Potential conflicts between item response theory and other sources of information, and their resolution, are described in the second section of the chapter, Part II.

The use of IRT models is now the 'gold standard' in PRO instrument development (Reise and Henson 2003; Nijsten 2012). IRT models have set in motion new rules of measurement particularly redefining reliability, item level-analysis, unidimensionality testing, scale scoring, among others. The increasing capacity and experience in IRT methodology at regulatory agencies such as the FDA coupled with user-friendly software, is further reducing the hurdles with applying IRT methodology in the context of registration trials. IRT models such as the Rasch model (RM) generate a linear metric scaled in logit units, representing the construct being measured, on which both the items and persons are located hierarchically reflecting their levels on the construct (Prieto et al. 2003). The probability of an item response for a given individual is then given by a logistic function of the difference between the item location and person location and nothing else (Twiss et al. 2011). These reflect the level of the underlying concept targeted by the item vis-a-vis that of the person, respectively. The parameters related to the item and person location are said to be invariant across samples (DeMars 2010).

'If it's not broken, why fix it'—why do we need new sophisticated analytics to explore psychometric properties of PROs when numerous tried and tested techniques based on classical test theory are available and serve the purpose?

P. Kamudoni et al., *Living with Chronic Disease: Measuring Important Patient-Reported Outcomes*, https://doi.org/10.1007/978-981-10-8414-0_5

Part I: Fine-Tuning of the HidroQoL Using Rasch Analysis

Key research questions:

- How well the prototype HidroQoL measure (~with 36 items) conformed to the Rasch model, particularly in terms of unidimensionality, whether targeting of the items to the population of hyperhidrosis patients was optimal and the functioning of response categories.
- Invariance/differential item functioning in the prototype HidroQoL measure across groups according to gender, age, site of hyperhidrosis and severity of disease.

Further, the analyses were utilised to identify need for and guide any content revision.

Methods

This study followed a prospective cross-sectional design. The major design consideration in Rasch analysis study is ensuring that respondents reflect the entire continuum of the construct, from the highest possible quality of life impairment and to the minimum possible impairment (Bond 2004). To ensure this, a large and heterogeneous patient population reflecting varying levels of disease severity and different types of hyperhidrosis is required. RM analyses can be carried out on a sample as small as 100. Nevertheless a sample size of at least 243 is large enough to achieve precision of ±0.5 logits within 99% level of confidence even in heavily skewed data (Linacre 1999). For stable estimation of category thresholds, at least ten observations are needed in each response category of an instrument. In view of this, the recruitment targeted 400 patients, representing the full range of disease severity according to the Hyperhidrosis Disease Severity Scale (HDSS).

Patients were recruited through hyperhidrosis online social networking communities, mainly the International Hyperhidrosis Society (IHHS) and the UK hyperhidrosis support group, from May to September 2012. A detailed description of the study population and procedures is available elsewhere (Kamudoni et al. 2015). Data analysis based on the Rasch model was carried out using RUMM 2030. Factor analysis was carried out using MPLUS-6 and STATA 11. A detailed description of the Rasch model and its application in scale development is available in Chap. 2.

As part of this study, patients completed the developmental HidroQoL. Rasch analyses were performed on the HidroQoL (36-item developmental HidroQoL) following item reduction using correlation analysis (see Chap. 6, page 118, Sect. 'Score Distribution, Correlation Analysis and Factor Analysis', for further details). Other data collected in the study included disease severity (using the HDSS), location of the hyperhidrosis and patient demographic characteristics.

Findings

Distribution of Responses

The basic patient characteristics for the sample used in this example are reported elsewhere (Kamudoni et al. 2015). The items showed a positive skew towards the higher response categories. All items except Q4, Q5, Q39, Q43 and Q45 had ceiling effects. In contrast, 13 items (Q4, Q5, Q13, Q16, Q19, Q25, Q38–Q41 and Q43–Q45) showed floor effects. Floor or ceiling effects are seen if either of the items extremities has at least 20% of responses (Both et al. 2007). Nevertheless, this did not compromise meaningful variability in the data, with 80% considered as the upper limit of endorsement for categories (Streiner and Norman 2008).

Three items (Q21, Q31 and Q35) had less than ten observations in the response category 'no, not at all'. This can be a problem in the context of Rasch modelling, particularly in estimating stable threshold values (Bond and Fox 2015). A general recommendation is to have a minimum of ten observations per category (Linacre 1999). There was no pattern to the missing data; thus data is missing at random. Nevertheless, the rates of missing data increase towards the end of the instrument.

Calibrating Item and Person Estimates

Rasch analysis was carried out on the HidroQoL-36. The likelihood ratio (LR) test for choice of appropriate RM supported the use of the partial credit model [−statistic = 529.47, df = 1.04, $p < 0.001$]. The partial credit model allows the differences between category thresholds of items to vary across items (Masters and Wright 1997). In this case, restricting such differences to be equal as assumed in the Rating Scale model might lead to a loss of information (Tennant and Conaghan 2007). Overall fit of the HidroQoL-36 to the RM based on the item-trait interaction chi-squared statistic (ITICS) and the mean fit residuals was poor [ITICS = 1642.32, df = 324, $p < 0.001$]. The item and person residual mean values reflected the same conclusion [item residual mean = 0.22, SD = 3.96; person residual mean = −0.00, SD = 1.48] (Appendix—Table 5.4, Analysis 1). Thus, although the items showed poor fit, the sample largely responded in conformity to the RM.

Model fit was also explored at the individual item and person level using fit residuals and ITICS. The fit residuals were between −2.5 and 2.5 (i.e. indicating optimal fit) for 15 items, greater than 2.5 (i.e. underfit) for 11 items and less than −2.5 (i.e. overfit) for 10 items. The underfitting group (fit residuals > 2.5) largely included items relevant to effects related to particular body areas. The over-fitting group (fit residuals < −2.5) primarily included items relating to negative emotions and the social impacts of hyperhidrosis, giving hints on the sources of the poor fit. Suboptimal response categorization is one cause of poor item fit to the RM (Linacre 1999). For an optimally functioning response categorisation, the choice of categories is expected to conform to the Rasch probabilistic pattern. Thus, functioning of the response categorisation for the HidroQoL was tested. Three items (Q8, Q29 and Q35) showed appropriately ordered category thresholds, where consecutive category thresholds increased with increasing levels of the latent variable (quality of life impact). The rest of the items had disordered thresholds, where the monotonicity of the thresholds was violated. This implies that for these items, response categories were used inconsistently, for example, respondents struggling to distinguish between response categories.

Measures applied in clinical practice need to be optimally targeted for the intended population (Pallant and Tennant 2007). The mean location parameters for persons and items were, therefore, compared. Furthermore, the spread of the items along the latent variable was also analysed. The mean person location was 0.5 (±0.82) in comparison to that of 0 (±0.6) for items.This indicates that the HidroQoL-36 was at a slightly lower level of HRQoL impairment in comparison to the sample. The item-person distribution map shows an even distribution of the items across the latent variable (Fig. 5.1). Reliability was assessed using the PSI. The HidroQoL-36 showed a PSI of 0.94, reflecting capability to distinguish up to four groups of QoL impairment levels. This is way more than the minimum levels needed for individual-level use.

Item Reduction and Refinement

Following the findings from the initial calibration of the HidroQoL-36, revisions were made to the HidroQoL-36 guided by the RM to address the category threshold disordering and then the misfit in the items. Subsequently, unidimensionality and local independence assumptions and the invariance property were tested.

Revising Item Response Scaling

Poorly functioning response options (i.e. disordered response category thresholds) may be addressed by combining/collapsing adjacent categories (Bond and Fox 2015). Rescoring of the HidroQoL response categories from 0-1-2-3 to 0-1-1-1-2 resolved disordering of category thresholds in all items as well as improving overall fit to the RM (Appendix Table 5.4, Analysis 2, 3; Appendix—Figs. 5.2a, b and 5.3).

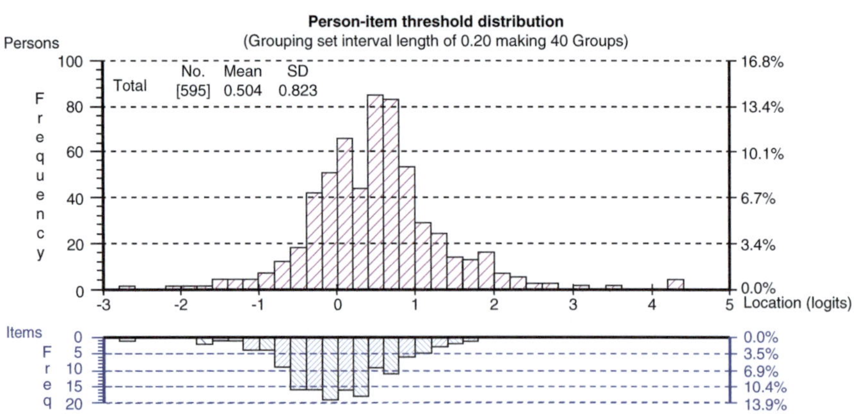

Fig. 5.1 Person-item distribution map of the HidroQoL-36 showing an even spread of the items across the latent variable

Removal of Misfitting Items

As a last resort, items with poor fit to the RM may need to be removed from an instrument due to the potential risk of bias on latent variables as well as item parameters (Baghaei 2008; Smith et al. 2008). Still, removal of items ought to consider the impact on the entire scale. Therefore, misfitting items were sequentially removed from the HidroQoL-36, iteratively assessing their impact on overall model fit as well as the remainder of the items, reliability of the instrument, and unidimensionality.

Four underfitting items, Q2, 'My choice of footwear is affected'; Q4, 'I have difficulties holding objects'; Q13, 'I find it hard to handle paper'; and Q43, 'My eyes feel irritated', relevant only to hyperhidrosis affecting particular body areas were the first candidates for removal. The ITICS declined to 768.26 (df = 288), reflecting improvement in fit (Appendix—Table 5.5, Analysis 4). Following further iterations of item reductions, 18 items showing good fit to the RM were achieved (Table 5.1).

The impact of removing items on the targeting of the HidroQoL against the sample was assessed by exploring the person-item distribution map. The difference between the person mean location and item mean location had increased ~from 0.87(±1.35) to 1.25 (±1.6) logits following item reduction (see Appendix—Table 5.5, Analysis 12). This is consistent with an increase in the number of persons with extreme scores (from 4 to 19 persons, following item reduction). Overall, the shift in the scale continuum and targeting is minimal (i.e. <0.5 logits).

Testing for Unidimensionality

The assumption of unidimensionality was formally tested for the HidroQoL-18 (~the PRO version following the first circle of item reduction). A principal component analysis (PCA) was carried out on the residuals of the Rasch model regression (i.e. after extraction of the target construct). The first component had an eigenvalue of 2 and accounted for 11.1% of variance in the residuals, which supported unidimensionality.

Further, a more stringent test of unidimensionality proposed by Smith (2002) was used. Person estimates generated from two pairs of item subsets, with the highest positive and negative loading above |±0.3| on the first principal component, respectively, were compared using a *t*-test. Items with high positive loadings included Q8, Q7, Q14, Q3 and Q15, while those with the highest negative loadings included Q29, Q22, Q37, Q47, Q35 and Q26. The proportion of significant *t*-tests was 5.3% [4.8%, 5.7%] confirming unidimensionality.

Analysis of Differential Item Functioning (DIF)

Invariance of item calibrations across populations and testing situations is considered as a key property of the RM (Reeve and Mâsse 2004). This means that when people with different demographic characteristics, such as females and males, complete an instrument, the scores obtained should not differ, holding the underlying latent variable constant. This property is formally assessed by testing individual items in a measure, for differential item functioning (DIF) across various demographic characteristics (see Chap. 2, Appendix: Technical Notes, Performing Rasch Analysis).

Table 5.1 Rasch model Parameter estimates for the final 18 items of the HidroQoL following item reduction

Fitting item		Location	SE	FitRes.	Chi-Sq	*p*-value	Threshold	
							1	2
Q3	My holidays are affected	0.47	0.09	−1.10	7.64	0.57	−1.70	1.70
Q7	My hobbies are affected	−0.01	0.09	0.83	5.31	0.81	−1.56	1.56
Q8	My physical activities are affected	−0.67	0.09	−1.30	4.41	0.88	−1.64	1.64
Q12	I avoid public speaking (e.g. presentations)	0.33	0.08	1.28	14.09	0.12	−0.97	0.97
Q14	My work is affected	0.51	0.09	−0.20	16.18	0.06	−1.74	1.74
Q15	My career decisions are affected (e.g. career choice)	0.49	0.08	−0.26	3.23	0.95	−0.81	0.81
Q18	I avoid meeting new people	1.16	0.08	0.07	3.03	0.96	−1.59	1.59
Q22	I feel nervous	−0.76	0.09	−1.80	16.52	0.06	−1.53	1.53
Q26	I feel frustrated	−1.08	0.09	−1.93	10.16	0.34	−1.42	1.42
Q29	Sweating is constantly on my mind	−1.04	0.09	−0.92	5.89	0.75	−2.00	2.00
Q32	My appearance is affected	−0.45	0.09	0.91	4.90	0.84	−1.55	1.55
Q34	I worry about leaving sweat marks on things	−1.07	0.09	1.40	9.02	0.44	−0.87	0.87
Q35	I worry about people's reactions	−2.05	0.10	−0.29	16.66	0.05	−2.40	2.40
Q37	I feel uncomfortable physically expressing affection (e.g. hugging others)	−0.03	0.09	−0.50	13.66	0.13	−1.65	1.65
Q38	My sex life is affected	1.60	0.08	1.19	14.60	0.10	−1.22	1.22
Q45	I worry about the additional chores in dealing with my condition	1.80	0.09	0.08	5.10	0.83	−1.74	1.74
Q47	I worry about my condition in future	0.17	0.08	0.38	8.12	0.52	−1.42	1.42
Q48	I find it hard to do things without planning in advance	0.63	0.08	−2.24	12.96	0.16	−1.43	1.43

The HidroQoL was assessed for DIF across various demographic characteristics (country, gender, age, body area affected, disease severity and comorbidity).

In total, six items showed DIF: items Q3, Q7, Q8, Q15, Q32 and Q34 showed uniform DIF for body area affected (Table 5.2). An illustration of uniform DIF in item Q8 (my physical activities are affected) is presented in Fig. 5.5. Item Q3 showed uniform DIF for disease severity; and item Q8 showed DIF for comorbidity. Finally, a set of 8 pure items without DIF for any of the patient characteristics considered were identified. In the final step, DIF was reassessed while anchoring the scale on the 'pure' set of items (Appendix—Table 5.6). There were no differences in the resultant items identified as showing DIF following the purification process.

DIF was non-trivial in all items affected. Item Q32 (my appearance is affected) was 3.3 logits easier for patients with generalised hyperhidrosis in comparison with the estimate based on all patients (Appendix—Table 5.7). This item was 2.06 logits more difficult for patients with palmar and plantar hyperhidrosis. DIF by age was most severe in item Q34: respondents in the age group 40 to 49 found this item was 2.9 logits easier than the average patient.

Various metrics suggested that the DIF observed in the items had no impact on the overall scale. Strong correlation was observed in the two sets of RM person estimates (i.e. from DIF-free items versus full instrument—with DIFd items (Pearson correlation = 0.94). Differences in sets of RM person estimates were <0.5 logits in 83.2% of the sample and <1 logit in 97.3%. T-test showed non-significant differences between RM person estimates ($p = 0.29$).

Table 5.2 DIF in items according to patient characteristics

	Age		Body area affected		Disease severity		Comorbidity	
Item	F-Stat.	*p*	F-Stat.	*p*	F-Stat.	*p*	F-Stat.	*p*
Q3	16.16	0.00002	12.7	0	7.48	0.000629		ns
Q7	1.55	ns	5.9	0.000571		ns		ns
Q8	14.5	0.00005	12.7	0.000001		ns	4.8	0.000265
Q12	1.67	ns		ns		ns		ns
Q14	0.41	ns		ns		ns		ns
Q15	1.15	ns	5.9	0.000584		ns		ns
Q18		ns		ns		ns		ns
Q22		ns		ns		ns		ns
Q26		ns		ns		ns		ns
Q29		ns		ns		ns		ns
Q32	10.29	0.000001	28.21	0		ns		ns
Q34	11.74	0.00001	14.79	0.00001		ns		ns
Q35		ns		ns		ns		ns
Q37		ns		ns		ns		ns
Q38		ns		ns		ns		ns
Q45		ns		ns		ns		ns
Q47	6.25	0.000365		ns		ns		ns
Q48		ns		ns		ns		ns

Notes: *F-Stat* F-statistic, *p* *p*-value, *ns* not significant

TCCs for groups by age, body area affected and disease severity were largely invariant; nonetheless, the TCC for the site of hyperhidrosis showed marginal variance (still $\leq$0.5 logits) (Appendix—Fig. 5.6a–d).

Testing for Local Independence

The RM assumption of local independence requires that any set of items should not share any meaningful correlation, once the latent variable is accounted for (Embretson 1996; Baghaei 2008). This is assessed using residual correlations. Similar to DIF analysis, the size and practical implications of local dependence are not clear based on correlations alone; thus it is usually necessary to estimate the impact of local dependence.

The HidroQoL-18[1] was assessed for local independence. Four item pairs showed a correlation greater than 0.2: Q15–Q32, Q3–Q34, Q14–Q15 and Q7–Q8. Of these, item sets Q7–Q8 and Q14–Q15 had the largest response dependence at 1.18 logits and 0.826, respectively, while that of Q4–Q34 was trivial (0.182 logits; i.e. <0.5 logits).

In order to conform to the RM assumption of local independence, one of the items of a pair showing non-trivial local dependence may need to be removed[2]. Therefore, two items (Q15 and Q8) were sequentially removed to address this issue; and an additional item (Q48) was removed—due to misfit following removal of the initial two items (Appendix—Table 5.8, Analysis 2–4). To achieve overall fit of the HidroQoL-15 to the RM, 22 persons demonstrating misfit to the RM were removed from the sample (Table 5.8, Analysis 5).

Part II: Integrating and Using Different Types of Data During the Item Reduction Process—Dealing with Friction

The process of fine-tuning a PRO measure is an integral part of the measure development process—in ensuring well-performing items (those that add to measurement) are retained in final measure versions. Statistical methods such as correlation analysis, multivariate regression analysis and factor analysis may help in evaluating an item's measurement attributes but provide no concrete information on the relevance of the items for the patient. Thus, in addition to integrating different types of quantitative data in the process, evidence from qualitative data reflecting importance of different themes has to guide the process.

For the HidroQoL, the initial item reduction step used results from correlation analysis, i.e. possible content overlap was suspected where the items shared a strong level of correlation (Spearman's correlation > 0.8). In such cases, additional

[1] Eighteen items showing fit to the RM at this point

[2] Choice of the item to be removed may need to take into account various other considerations such as location of the item in the concept continuum and qualitative considerations.

considerations were made of the conceptual scope of each item, as well as the importance of the issue addressed. For example, the items 'my self-confidence is affected' and 'my self-esteem is affected' were highly correlated. The self-confidence item was more prevalent during the qualitative study, making it the preferred item. Relative to other techniques, this approach is straight forward and is more transparent than the other methods. Thus even where other methods are planned, correlation analysis may be easily integrated as a first step. Thirteen items were removed from the HidroQoL, leaving 36 items (HidroQoL-36).

Further item reduction of the HidroQoL was carried out based on results of EFA (see Chap. 6). Iterations of EFA analyses were performed on the HidroQoL-36 until a simple structure was achieved, i.e. where each item predominantly loaded to a single factor and had negligible/insignificant loading on any additional factors. Items which were not loading to any factor or cross-loading on multiple factors were removed, taking into account their content (content relevance). Although a one-factor as well as two-factor solution was supported by the results, a two-factor solution offered more insight into the nature of hyperhidrosis impacts. Moreover, the two factors were interpretable as impact on daily life activities and psychosocial impact.

Rasch analysis was carried out on the HidroQoL-36. Performing the analysis on this version of the HidroQoL ensured comparability with the EFA as well as guaranteed that the first stage of item reduction still incorporated qualitative consideration from the correlation analysis-based item reduction. Items showing poor fit to the RM were iteratively identified and removed, taking into account impacts on content validity, impairment continuum covered by the scale and impact on the reliability during each iteration. This provided thorough insights into the contribution of each item to the conceptual definition of the target concept. Analysis using the Rasch model allowed the conceptualisation of HRQoL assessed by the HidroQoL as a construct relevant to all types of hyperhidrosis.

The integration of two frameworks—EFA and IRT (Rasch model)—was important, for cross-validating results, as well as to gain additional insights into the measure, based on the slightly different perspectives on the measurement model underpinned by these approaches. In the RA, for example, all hyperhidrosis-site-specific item showed poor fit suggesting that they were not assessing the same Rasch latent variable (hyperhidrosis-QoL). During the EFA these items all belonged to a single factor. The EFA, however, would not indicate whether this factor was part and parcel of a broad QoL construct relevant for all forms of hyperhidrosis or not. If a modular approach to measure development was taken, such items could have been used to create site-specific modules.

Although the Rasch analysis and EFA produced slightly different instruments, 11 items were common. The major difference was in items assessing the psychosocial impact domain. One reason for this might be the fact that the Rasch model assesses whether an item is used consistently, in line with Rasch probabilistic conditions, i.e. whether patients with greater impairment have a higher probability of a higher score than those with a lower impairment (Tennant et al. 2004). Furthermore, the RM conceptualises the latent variable as a linear metric measuring the latent variable/construct from a low to high severity level, with items placed hierarchically on the metric according to their level of difficulty (Pallant and Tennant 2007). In contrast, the FA linear model does not accommodate the latent variable's severity dimension; it makes no consideration of item difficulty and thus lacks the capability to deal with item redundancy. Since FA assesses items based on shared covariation, those where this is low may be penalised despite their contribution to overall scale, for example, the item 'My sex life is affected'.

The final version of the HidroQoL utilised the taxonomy from the EFA to provide two subscales, impact on daily life activities and psychosocial impact, in addition to the overall scale. The choice of items was based on the Rasch analysis, in order to simultaneously take into account the entire continuum of impairment in HRQoL and realise a unidimensional construct. Three items were added on the 15 selected based on RA optimisation, 'my physical activities are affected', 'I feel embarrassed' and my choice of clothing is affected'. The first two were included in the FA-reduced instrument. Although the RM showed some response dependence between the item 'my physical activities are affected' and 'my hobbies are affected', the two items represent separate and mutually exclusive concepts. The items 'I feel embarrassed' and 'my choice of clothing is affected' emerged as the most prevalent themes during qualitative research; thus their omission might have negatively impacted content validity and applicability of the instrument. Thus the process of selecting items for the final version of the HidroQoL and the development of a measurement model explicitly addressed the friction between the qualitative and quantitative methods as well as between the classical test theory and modern test theories, applied in this study. The most statistically viable measurement model was implemented, but not at the neglect of the priorities of patients.

Concluding Remarks

In her commentary, Embretson (1996) argued that modern test theory introduces new rules to measurement which are fundamentally different from rules represented under the traditional/classical test theory (CTT). Therefore, rather than replacing CTT, integration of modern test into instrument development offers additional insights on measures' capabilities—such integrated frameworks are the new gold standard in PRO instrument development.

This chapter has presented an example of how modern test theory (such as the Rasch model) may be used in refining a PRO measure, particularly in assessing attributes which may not be easily explored within traditional/classical test theory such as assessing response category functioning and differential item functioning.

The Rasch model is based on the premise that the probability of a particular response on an item is driven by the difference between the item location and person location on a common metric measuring the underlying concept and nothing else. This allows the hierarchical ordering of items on a hypothetical severity continuum of the underlying concept being measured by an instrument (e.g. HRQoL impairment). In general, the Rasch model is relevant for unidimensional concepts and is based on the assumptions of unidimensionality and local independence. Advances in item response theory have brought models that can handle multidimensional concepts.

The Rasch model (as well as other IRT models) may be utilised to assess various attributes for PRO measures such as unidimensionality, local independence, optimal functioning of response categorisation, differential item functioning and targeting of a PRO measure to a sample. This may facilitate fine-tuning of new measure as well as item reduction.

For example, lack of overall model fit of a PRO measure to the Rasch model may indicate that hierarchical ordering of the items on the latent concept continuum is not invariant across the different levels of impairment (Pallant and Tennant 2007).

Poor item fit to the model may suggest that an item measures a different construct other than the one being measured by the Rasch model—the target concept of a PRO. Removal of misfitting items may be necessary to achieve overall good fit to the Rasch model. Thus, to support item reduction, misfitting items may be removed from the model/instrument, sequentially. In turn, the impact of removing such items on the scope and range of the continuum of the latent variable, reliability and increase in extreme scores (ceiling/floor effects) can be explored.

Because the Rasch model does not distinguish between items and person in calculations, it is also possible to assess how well a given sample fits the model. This may be useful in identifying certain response patterns, e.g. 'lucky guessing' or 'carelessness', which may facilitate refining of the validation sample.

In the case study presented in this chapter, the Rasch model was used to fine-tune the HidroQoL measure:

Response category threshold results were used to reduce response options of the HidroQoL from a 5-point Likert scale to a 3-point Likert scaling.

Invariance/DIF was assessed for patient groups based on age, disease severity and comorbidity. Although eight items showed DIF, this was considered to have non-significant impact on the total score; therefore no item was removed based on that.

Following revisions (i.e. collapsing of response categories and removal of misfitting items), the final version of the HidroQoL showed unidimensionality.

The items showed appropriate targeting, i.e. based on comparison of the severity of HRQoL impairment assessed/targeted by the items versus that of the sample.

The items appeared to be evenly spread along the HRQoL impairment continuum—indicating that the measure was well designed in terms of assessing HRQoL impairment across different levels.

Although it might be possible to assess some of the attributes explored using other techniques (such as traditional psychometrics)—e.g. unidimensionality or differential item functioning—the credibility, transparency and ease with which these are undertaken using the Rasch model make the Rasch (or item response theory) a preferred approach where this is feasible.

Appendix

Responses to the HidroQoL Items

Table 5.3 Distribution of the HidroQoL item scores

Item	Descriptor	No, not at all		A little		Somewhat		Quite a bit		Very much		Missing	
		n	%	*n*	%	*n*	%	n	%	*n*	%	*n*	%
Q1	My choice of clothing is affected	18	3	30	5	51	9	110	18	386	65	0	0
Q2	My choice of footwear is affected	106	18	38	6	66	11	72	12	313	53	0	0
Q3	My holidays are affected (e.g. planning, activities)	70	12	67	11	143	24	121	20	194	33	0	0
Q4	I have difficulties holding objects	201	34	71	12	96	16	112	19	115	19	0	0
Q5	I have difficulties handling money	262	44	71	12	102	17	79	13	81	14	0	0
Q6	I find it hard to touch other people	98	16	43	7	67	11	89	15	298	50	0	0
Q7	My hobbies are affected	52	9	51	9	95	16	153	26	244	41	0	0
Q8	My physical activities are affected	29	5	52	9	77	13	129	22	308	52	0	0
Q9	My outdoor activities are affected	30	5	52	9	81	14	110	18	322	54	0	0
Q10	My summer activities are affected	21	4	37	6	67	11	96	16	374	63	0	0
Q11	My everyday housework is affected	107	18	89	15	127	21	124	21	148	25	0	0
Q12	I avoid public speaking (e.g. presentations)	84	14	75	13	72	12	96	16	268	45	0	0
Q13	I find it hard to handle paper	193	32	49	8	69	12	91	15	193	32	0	0
Q14	My work is affected	65	11	60	10	132	22	149	25	189	32	0	0
Q15	My career decisions are affected (e.g. career choice)	107	18	49	8	69	12	111	19	259	44	0	0
Q16	I have difficulties using touch technologies (e.g. computer keyboard, smart phones)	198	33	47	8	90	15	105	18	155	26	0	0
Q17	I do not socialise as much as I would like to	60	10	69	12	98	16	113	19	255	43	0	0
Q18	I avoid meeting new people	117	20	75	13	114	19	138	23	148	25	3	1
Q19	I avoid going out	135	23	88	15	118	20	133	22	118	20	3	1
Q20	My personal relationships are affected	89	15	87	15	139	23	120	20	157	26	3	1

Q21	I feel embarrassed	9	2	15	3	44	7	89	15	435	73	3	1
Q22	I feel nervous	30	5	35	6	70	12	126	21	331	56	3	1
Q23	I feel hopeless	110	18	73	12	95	16	79	13	235	39	3	1
Q24	I feel sad	117	20	109	18	99	17	79	13	188	32	3	1
Q25	I feel depressed	152	26	115	19	102	17	66	11	157	26	3	1
Q26	I feel frustrated	22	4	42	7	61	10	99	17	367	62	4	1
Q27	My self-confidence is affected	28	5	51	9	81	14	117	20	314	53	4	1
Q28	My self-esteem is affected	47	8	51	9	78	13	110	18	305	51	4	1
Q29	Sweating is constantly on my mind	17	3	47	8	70	12	146	25	311	52	4	1
Q30	I avoid taking on new challenges	93	16	77	13	131	22	118	20	172	29	4	1
Q31	I feel self-conscious	9	2	27	5	50	8	108	18	397	67	4	1
Q32	My appearance is affected	33	6	52	9	95	16	113	19	298	50	4	1
Q33	I worry about my body odour	102	17	98	16	105	18	105	18	181	30	4	1
Q34	I worry about leaving sweat marks on things	30	5	35	6	49	8	82	14	395	66	4	1
Q35	I worry about people's reactions	7	1	27	5	58	10	126	21	370	62	7	1
Q36	I find it hard to be near other people	79	13	69	12	129	22	136	23	175	29	7	1
Q37	I feel uncomfortable physically expressing affection (e.g. hugging others)	49	8	57	10	103	17	135	23	243	41	8	1
Q38	My sex life is affected	172	29	92	15	128	22	67	11	125	21	11	2
Q39	My choice of food and drinks is affected	260	44	88	15	108	18	58	10	71	12	10	2
Q40	I feel uncomfortable in my shoes	138	23	70	12	66	11	89	15	223	37	9	2
Q41	I have problems with being barefooted	188	32	49	8	38	6	61	10	251	42	8	1
Q42	My skin feels uncomfortable	83	14	69	12	99	17	113	19	221	37	10	2
Q43	My eyes feel irritated	305	51	72	12	87	15	61	10	59	10	11	2
Q44	I worry about the additional money spent in dealing with my condition	173	29	130	22	105	18	75	13	101	17	11	2
Q45	I worry about the additional chores in dealing with my condition	155	26	126	21	103	17	110	18	94	16	7	1
Q46	I worry about the additional time spent in dealing with my condition	119	20	108	18	116	19	111	19	131	22	10	2
Q47	I worry about my condition in future	61	10	61	10	77	13	144	24	244	41	8	1
Q48	I find it hard to do things without planning in advance	90	15	64	11	112	19	117	20	204	34	8	1
Q49	My whole life is affected	23	4	52	9	71	12	118	20	321	54	10	2

Iterative Steps in the Item Reduction Process of the HidroQoL and Rasch Model Fit Statistics

Table 5.4 Overall model fit statistics for the 36 items HidroQoL and subsequent versions after rescoring

Action	Overall model fit			Item fit residuals		Person fit residuals		Dimensionality	PSI
	Chi	df	*p*	Mean	SD	Mean	SD	Sign. t-test(%)	
1. All 36 items included	1642.64	324	0.00	0.22	3.96	−0.01	1.5	26.39%[a]	0.94
2. Revise scoring to 01123	1404.5	324	0.00	0.00	3.9	−0.089	1.55	33.28%[b]	0.94
3. Revise scoring to 01113	1087.4	324	0.001	−0.05	3.48	−0.234	1.64	28.57%	0.94

[a]Items 13, 4, 2, 6, 7, 42 and 34 had positive loadings of 0.3 and above. Items 29, 18, 26, 20, 48, 36, 32, 30, 17, 21, 24 and 27 had negative loadings

[b]Items 13, 4, 2, 6, 7, 42 and 34 had positive loadings of 0.3 and above. Items 26, 35, 18, 29, 22, 48, 32, 20, 17, 36, 21, 30, 24, 36 and 27 had negative loadings below—0.3

Table 5.5 The item reduction procedure—impact of item reduction steps on overall fit of overall model and individual items

Action	Overall model fit			Item fit residuals		Person fit residuals		PSI	Fit resid >2.5	Fit resid < −2.5
	Chi	df	p	Mean	SD	Mean	SD			
3. Revise scoring to 01113	1087.40	324.00	0.001	−0.05	3.48	−0.23	1.64	0.94	39, 2, 13, 43, 33, 11, 4	26, 20, 22, 17, 30, 24, 27, 36
4. Q2, Q4, Q13 and Q43 removed	768.26	288.00	0.001	−0.12	3.35	−0.31	1.59	0.94	39, 6, 11, 33, 42, 1, 44	22, 20, 24, 17, 30, 27, 36
5. Q39, Q6 and Q11 removed	612.89	261.00	0.001	−0.29	2.69	−0.35	1.55	0.93	33, 42, 1, 44	20, 24, 17, 30, 27, 36
6. Q36, Q27 and Q30	453.34	234.00	0.001	−0.22	2.26	−0.34	1.48	0.92	33, 42, 1, 44	22, 20, 24, 17
7. Q33 and Q42 removed	346.51	216.00	0.001	−0.23	1.96	−0.34	1.43	0.92	44, 1	24, 20, 17
8. Q17 and Q20 removed	290.29	198.00	0.001	−0.21	1.78	−0.33	1.37	0.91	44, 1	21, 24
9. Item 1 deleted	277.60	189.00	0.001	−0.23	1.68	−0.34	1.37	0.91	44	21, 24
10. Q24 deleted	233.68	180.00	0.001	−0.19	1.54	−0.34	1.35	0.90	44	–
11. Q44 deleted	239.49	171.00	0.001	−0.27	1.39	−0.34	1.33	0.89	–	21
12. Q21 deleted	194.00	162.00	0.04	−0.25	1.22	−0.33	1.37	0.89		
13. Six respondents removed	178.49	162.00	0.18	−0.25	1.16					
14. Six respondents removed	169.57	162.00	0.33	−0.25	1.14	−0.31	1.30	0.89		
15. Two respondents removed	171.47	162.00	−0.25	−0.25	1.13	−0.31	1.29	0.89		

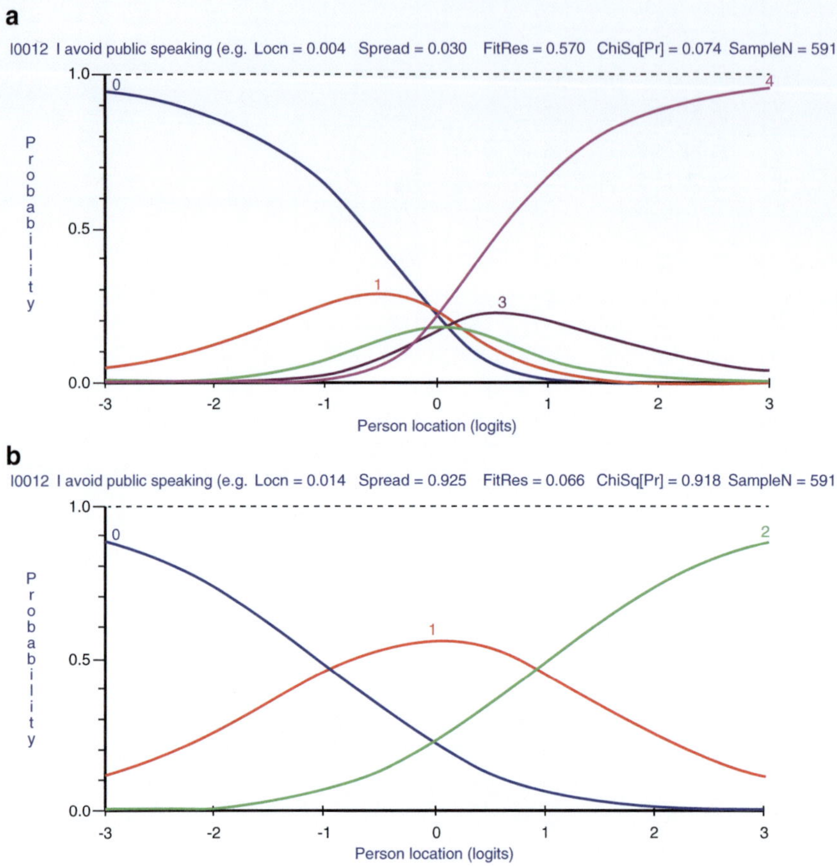

Fig. 5.2 An illustration of the impact of rescoring on category probability curves. (**a**) Item 12 (I avoid public speaking) showing disordered category probability curves, prior to rescoring. (**b**) Item 12 (I avoid public speaking) showing appropriately ordered category probability curves after rescoring from 5 to 3 categories

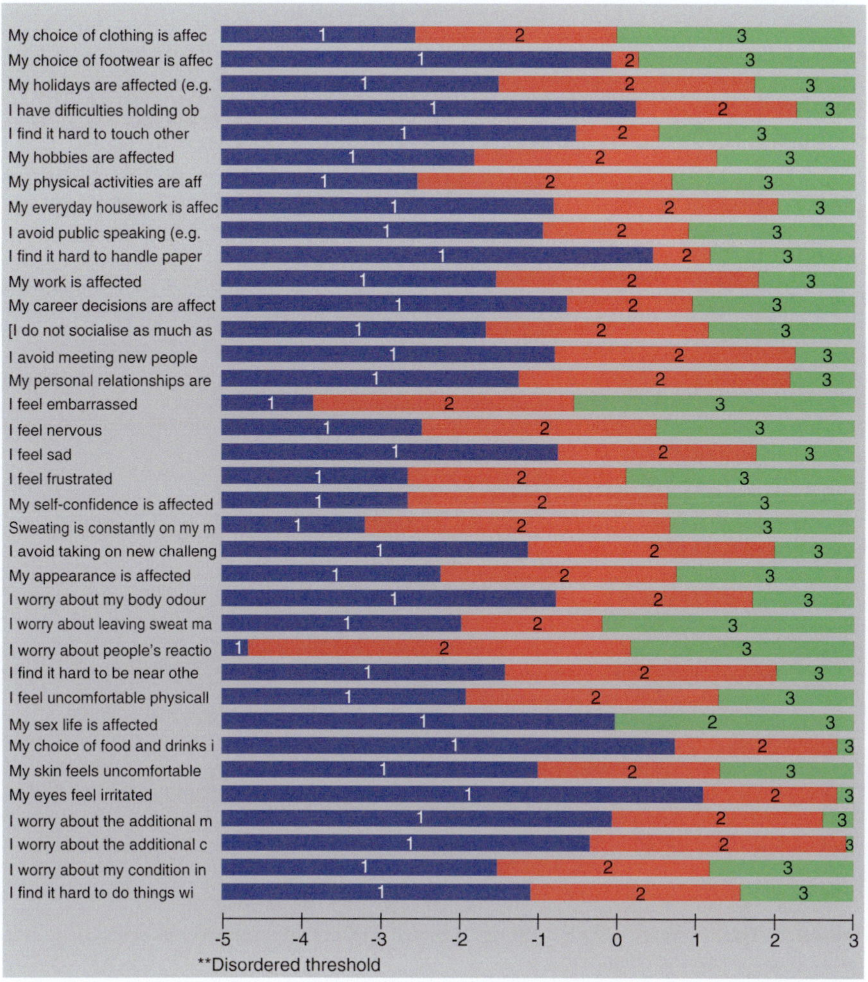

Fig. 5.3 Item threshold map of the HidroQoL-36 after rescoring to 3-point response categories

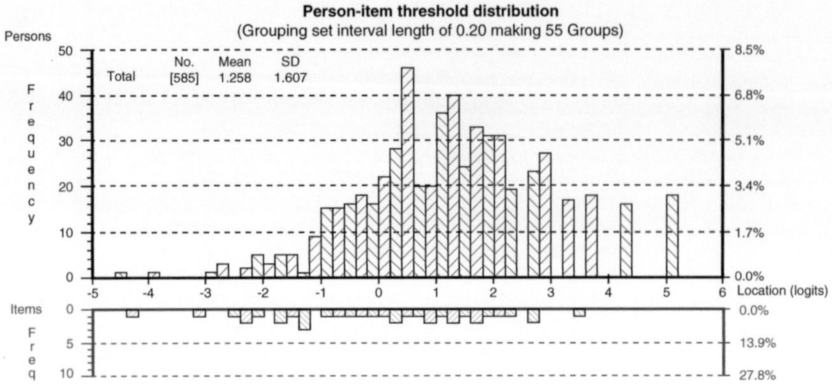

Fig. 5.4 Person-item distribution showing targeting of the HidroQoL-18 following item reduction

Evaluation of Differential Item Functioning

Table 5.6 Pure set of items showing no DIF following the purification

	Location	Threshold_1	Threshold_2
Q7	−0.498	−1.554	1.554
Q14	−0.010	−1.700	1.700
Q18	0.607	−1.536	1.536
Q29	−1.513	−1.983	1.983
Q37	−0.511	−1.634	1.634
Q38	1.061	−1.226	1.226
Q45	1.222	−1.750	1.750
Q47	−0.359	−1.417	1.417

Table 5.7 The magnitude of DIF in the developmental HidroQoL: comparisons across body area affected, age group and comorbidity

Body area affected			Age group			Comorbidity		
Item	Difficulty estimate	DIF size	Item	Difficulty estimate	DIF size	Item	Difficulty estimate	DIF size
Q3_original	−0.06							
Q3_head	0.00	−0.06	Q3_18 to 29	1.60	−1.66			
Q3_axilar	1.31	−1.36	Q3_30 to 39	0.95	−1.01			
Q3_generic	0.22	−0.28	Q3_40 to 49	0.73	−0.78			
Q3_p&f	1.23	−1.29	Q3_50+	−0.06	0.01			
Q8_Original	−1.13							
Q8_head	−0.79	−0.34	Q8_18 to 29	−0.13	−1.00	Q8_none	0.07	−1.20

Table 5.7 (continued)

Body area affected			Age group			Comorbidity		
Item	Difficulty estimate	DIF size	Item	Difficulty estimate	DIF size	Item	Difficulty estimate	DIF size
Q8_axilar	0.22	−1.35	Q8_30 to 39	0.26	−1.39	Q8_ men	−4.51	3.38
Q8_ generic	−0.70	−0.43	Q8_40 to 49	−0.24	−0.89	Q8_ diab	−1.21	0.08
Q8_p&f	−0.38	−0.75	Q8_50 to 59	−1.36	0.23	Q8_ hyper	−1.28	0.15
Q12_ original	−0.21							
Q12_head	0.64	−0.84						
Q12_ axilar	0.24	−0.44						
Q12_ generic	0.36	−0.57						
Q12_p&f	1.21	−1.42						
Q32 original	−0.97							
Q32_head	−1.76	0.79	Q32_18 to 29	0.60	−1.57			
Q32_ axilar	−0.28	−0.69	Q32_30 to 39	−0.50	−0.47			
Q32_ generic	−4.25	3.28	Q32_40 to 49	−0.11	−0.86			
Q32_p&f	1.09	−2.06	Q32_50+	−0.67	−0.30			
Q34_ Original	−1.53							
Q34_head	0.14	−1.67	Q34_18 to 29	−1.86	0.33			
Q34_ axilar	−1.14	−0.38	Q34_18 to 29	−0.79	−0.74			
Q34_ generic	−0.88	−0.65	Q34_40 to 49	−4.42	2.89			
Q34_p&f	−4.49	2.96	Q34_50 to 59	−0.12	−1.40			
Q48_ original	0.09							
Q48_head	0.68	−0.59						
Q48_ axilar	1.20	−1.10						
Q48_ generic	0.31	−0.22						
Q48_p&f	1.42	−1.32						

Note: Size of DIF for each item is [item difficulty estimate, whole sample (Qxx_original)—group-specific item estimate]

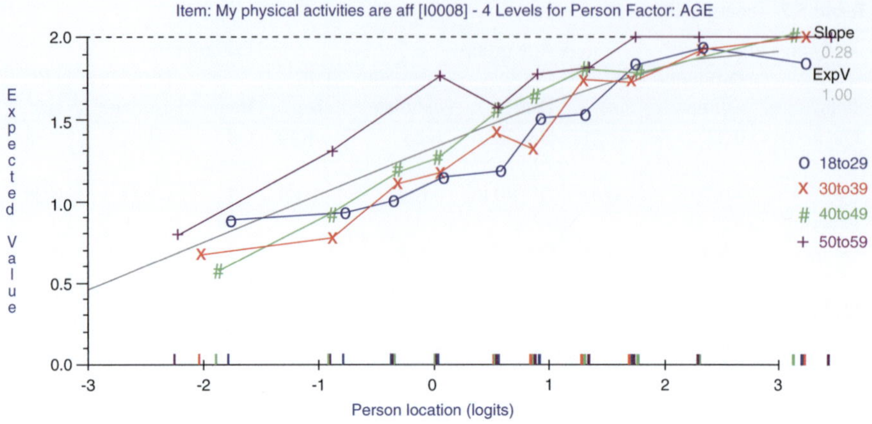

Fig. 5.5 An illustration of DIF as reflected in empirical group-specific item characteristic curves—ICC—for item Q8 (my physical activities are affected) showing expected score for each level of the latent variable traced for each age group

Analysis of DIF Impact at Scale Level: Comparison of Test Characteristic Curves (TCCs) of the HidroQoL-18 Across Patient Subgroups

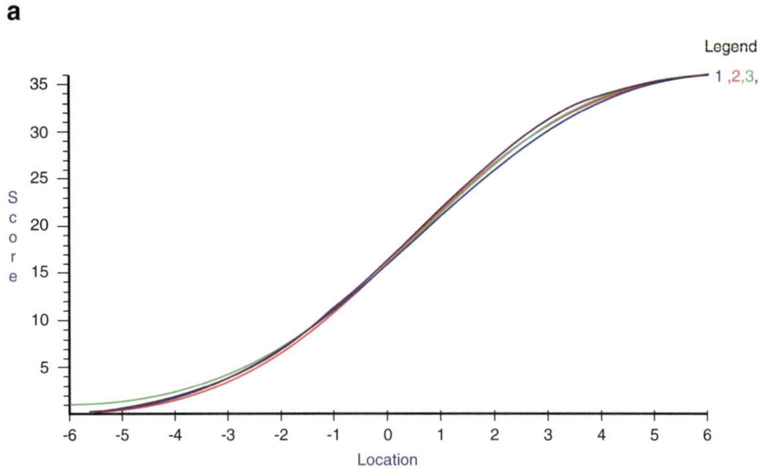

Fig. 5.6 Test characteristic curves for the HidroQoL-18. (**a**) *TCCs by age.* (**b**) *TCCs by body area affected.* (**c**) *TCCs by severity of disease.* (**d**) *TCCs by comorbidity*

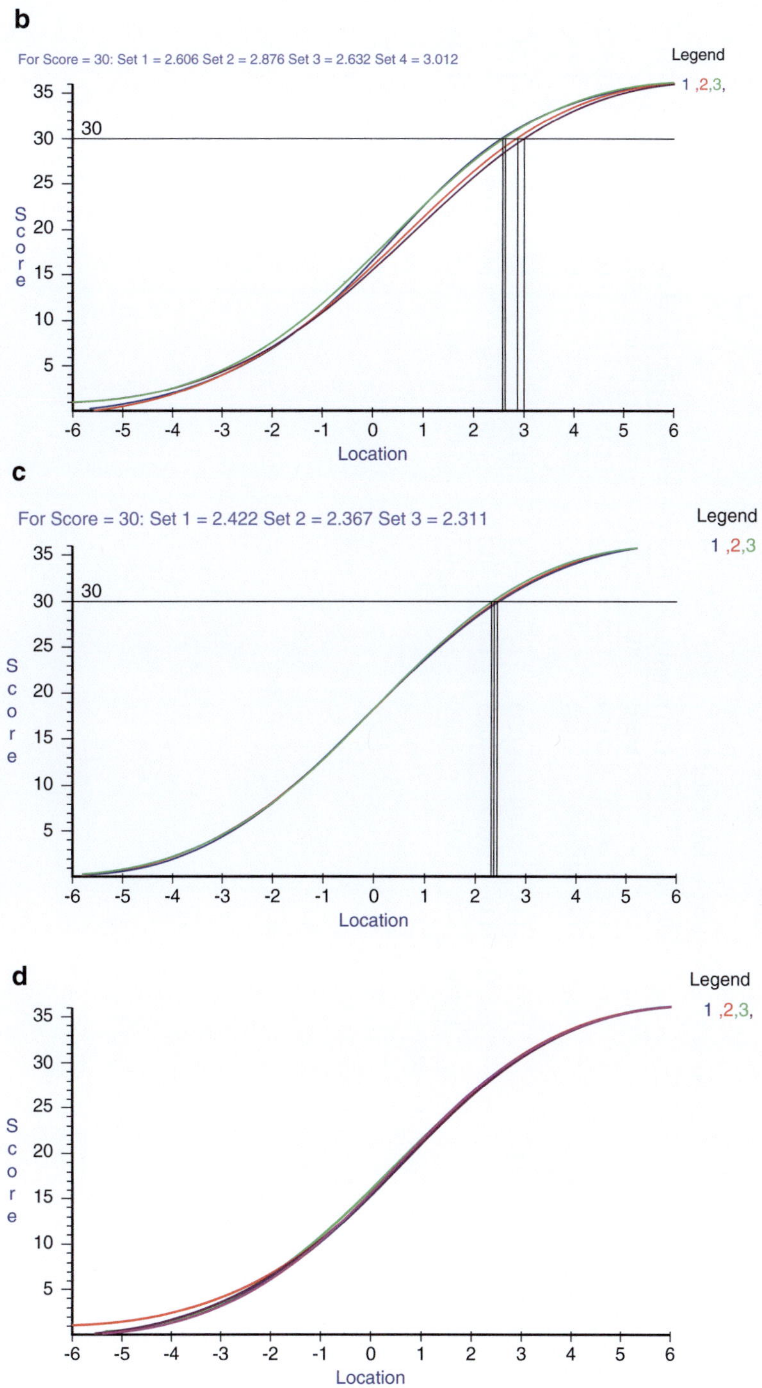

Fig. 5.6 (continued)

Local Dependence

Table 5.8 Impact of adjusting for response dependence on overall model fit

Action	Overall model fit			Item fit residuals		Person fit residuals		Person location		Unid	PSI
	Chi	Df	*p*	Mean	SD	Mean	SD	Mean	SD	Sig test(%)	
1. Splitting Q7, Q15 and Q3	267.93	188	<0.001	−0.29	1.29	−0.3	1.18	1.1	1.66		0.872
2. Removing item 15, from HidroQoL-18	168.94	153	0.179	−0.27		−0.3	1.24	1.3	1.67		0.882
3. Removing Q8 from HidroQoL	187.96	144	<0.001	−0.23	1.33	−0.3	1.2	1.31	1.68		0.88
4. Removing Q48	165.72	135	0.039	−0.2	1.21	−0.3	1.18	1.34	1.66	7.09	
5. Removing 22 persons	159.64	135	0.07	−0.09	1.19	−0.24	1.05	1.365	1.65	3.42	0.869

Note: *Chi* chi-squared; *df* degrees of freedom

References

Baghaei P (2008) The Rasch model as a construct validation tool. Rasch Meas Trans 22(1):1145–1146

Both H et al (2007) Critical review of generic and dermatology-specific health-related quality of life instruments. J Invest Dermatol 127:2726–2739

Bond T (2004) Validity and assessment: a Rasch measurement perspective. Metodología Las Cienc Comport 5:179–194

Bond TG, Fox CM (2015) Applying the Rasch model: fundamental measurement in the human sciences. Routledge, Abingdon

Coste J, Guillemin F, Pouchot J, Fermanian J (1997) Methodological approaches to shortening composite measurement scales. J Clin Epidemiol 50:247–252

DeMars C (2010) Item response theory. Oxford University Press, Oxford. http://books.google.co.uk/books?id=KOADeYBt7sIC

Embretson SE (1996) The new rules of measurement. Psychol Assess 8(4):341

Kamudoni P, Mueller B, Salek MS (2015) The development and validation of a disease-specific quality of life measure in hyperhidrosis: the hyperhidrosis quality of life index (HidroQOL©). Qual Life Res 24(4):1017–1027

Linacre JM (1999) Investigating rating scale category utility. J Outcome Meas 3(2):103

Masters NG, Wright DB (1997) Handbook of modern item response theory. In: Linden WJ, Hambleton RK (eds) The partial credit model. Springer, New York, NY, pp 101–121. https://doi.org/10.1007/978-1-4757-2691-6_6

Nijsten T (2012) Dermatology life quality index: time to move forward. J Investig Dermatol 132(1):11–13

Nijsten T, Unaeze J, Stern R (2006) Refinement and reduction of the impact of psoriasis questionnaire: classical test theory vs. Rasch analysis. Br J Dermatol 154:692–700

Pallant JF, Tennant A (2007) An introduction to the Rasch measurement model: an example using the hospital anxiety and depression scale (HADS). Br J Clin Psychol 46(1):1–18

Prieto L, Alonso J, Lamarca R (2003) Classical test theory versus Rasch analysis for quality of life questionnaire reduction. Health Qual Life Outcomes 1(1):27

Reeve BB, Hays RD, Chang CH, Perfetto EM (2007) Applying item response theory to enhance health outcomes assessment. Qual Life Res 16:1–3

Reeve BB, Mâsse LC (2004) Methods for testing and evaluating survey questionnaires. In: Presser S, Rothgeb JM, Couper MP, Lessler JT, Martin E, Martin J, Singer E (eds) Item response theory modeling for questionnaire evaluation. John Wiley & Sons, Inc., Hoboken, NJ, pp 247–273. https://doi.org/10.1002/0471654728.ch13

Reise SP, Henson JM (2003) A discussion of modern versus traditional psychometrics as applied to personality assessment scales. J Pers Assess 81(2):93–103

Reise SP, Haviland MG (2005) Item response theory and the measurement of clinical change. J Pers Assess 84(3):228–238

Smith AB, Rush R, Fallowfield LJ, Velikova G, Sharpe M (2008) Rasch fit statistics and sample size considerations for Polytomous data. BMC Med Res Methodol 8(1):33

Smith EV (2002) Detecting and evaluating the impact of multidimensionality using item fit statistics and principal component analysis of residuals. J Appl Meas 3(2):205–231

Streiner DL, Norman GR (2008) Health measurement Scales : a practical guide to their development and use. Oxford University Press, Oxford. http://books.google.co.uk/books?id=UbKijeRqndwC

Tennant A, Conaghan PG (2007) The Rasch measurement model in rheumatology: what is it and why use it? When should it be applied, and what should one look for in a Rasch paper? Arthritis Care Res 57(8):1358–1362

Tennant A et al (2004) Application of Rasch analysis in the development and application of quality of life instruments. Value Health 7(Suppl 1):S22–S26

Twiss J, Meads DM, Preston EP, Crawford SR, McKenna SP (2011) Can we rely on the dermatology life quality index as a measure of the impact of psoriasis or atopic dermatitis. J Investig Dermatol 132(1):76–84

Assessing the Performance of PRO Measures Against Expectations: Psychometric Evaluation

6

Evaluating construct validity involves assessing the extent to which theoretically derived hypotheses relating to the construct being measured by an instrument are supported by empirical evidence (Terwee et al. 2007). Although there is no prescription regarding type, form and nature of such empirical evidence, the need to demonstrate construct validity arises each time a measure is used in a new situation or where different inference will be drawn, reflecting on the continuous nature of the validation process (Streiner and Norman 2008). For this reason, there is an even greater imperative to generate such evidence for new instruments.

Following the qualitative instrument development steps addressed in previous chapters, quantitative empirical evidence from several studies and analyses is assembled to evaluate inferences in a defined context of use, i.e. to assess psychometric properties. This chapter will illustrate how classical test theory (CTT) approaches are used to achieve using studies carried out in the development of the HidroQoL as an example. Specifically, the focus of the chapter is on how well the measure's scores function as expected (construct validity), understanding of measurement error associated with the measure scores (reliability assessment), ability of scores to capture change in the patient's condition longitudinally and exploring criteria for clinically meaningful interpretation of scores.

This chapter describes the different types of studies and analyses that might be useful for testing the psychometric attributes of a new PRO measure—representing Step 8 of the new PROs roadmap—generating psychometric evidence and other supportive information. Research carried out as part of the validation procedures for the HidroQoL to assess reliability, construct validity, responsiveness and interpretability will be used as a case study, to illustrate the process and practical aspects involved in this step.

P. Kamudoni et al., *Living with Chronic Disease: Measuring Important Patient-Reported Outcomes*, https://doi.org/10.1007/978-981-10-8414-0_6

Part I: Assessing the Construct Validity of the HidroQoL

In this section, we will illustrate the steps involved in establishing the accuracy and credibility of the PRO measures. Initially, the measurement model (internal structure) of the HidroQoL was explored, while also performing item reduction—to remove items not contributing to the measurement model. Further, various hypothesis tests were carried out in assessing the known group validity, convergent validity and the HidroQoL scores:

Score distribution, correlation analysis and factor analysis—aims at understanding the measurement characteristics of the scale such as the distribution of item scores, relationships among items and the underlying internal structure of measure. For a well-functioning tool, it is expected that:

Criteria 1: responses should be evenly spread across response options, i.e. the extreme ends (ceiling and floor) should not account for more than 15% of the sample.

Criteria 2: individual items should not have a strong correlation, i.e. correlation >0.08 indicates multicollinearity (Fayers and Machin 2007a, b).

Criteria 3: items are properly loaded in EFA test suggesting 'no Items' with (1) highest loading below 0.4; (2) more than one loading above 0.4, with none above 0.5; (3) residual variance (uniqueness) of 0.7 or more; and (4) content mismatch with their factors (Lackey et al. 2003; Costello and Osborne 2005; Nijsten et al. 2006).

Known group validity—aims at capturing the group differences in scores across a 'hypothesised/expected' category. It is expected that the HidroQoL should differentiate between disease severities and location of the disease.

Hypothesis 1: Patients with more severe disease would report lower HidroQoL scores.
Hypothesis 2: Patients with disease that involves more areas of the body would have lower HidroQoL scores.

Convergent validity—aimed at capturing the association between scores of the HidroQoL and those of other related established instruments. In some cases, this can also involve testing 'lack of' association with measures assessing concepts that are not related; this is called divergent validities. The relationship between the scores of the HidroQoL and other measures of disease impact was assessed. This included EQ-5D score, DLQI score, HDSS score and an item assessing daily time spent managing condition.

Hypothesis 1: The HidroQoL score is positively correlated with patient's HDSS score.
Hypothesis 2: Patient's HidroQoL score was positively correlated with the DLQI score.

Hypothesis 3: The HidroQoL scores are not correlated with EQ-5Ds 'mobility' and 'self-care' domain scores.

Hypothesis 4: The HidroQoL scores are correlated with EQ-5D-5L domains on 'usual activities', 'anxiety/depression' and 'pain or discomfort'.

Hypothesis 5: Greater impairment in quality of life is associated with more time spent in managing the condition.

Methods

Study Design

The construct validity of the HidroQoL was tested in two studies. Participants in both studies included members of hyperhidrosis patient's groups—International Hyperhidrosis Society (IHHS) and UK hyperhidrosis support group—with all types of hyperhidrosis and across all severity levels. Eligibility criteria included self-reported hyperhidrosis, age of 18 years or above, Hyperhidrosis Disease Severity Scale (HDSS) score greater than 1 and onset of hyperhidrosis in teenage years or early adult years.

The first study (study 1) followed a cross-sectional design where respondents completed the developmental HidroQoL questionnaire on a single assessment. In addition, data were also collected on the Hyperhidrosis Disease Severity Score, patient demographics, characteristics of disease and treatment-related characteristics. The score distribution, correlation analysis and factor analysis were assessed in this study.

The second study (study 2) followed a longitudinal design with two follow-up assessments (at baseline/day 1, day 7 and day 21). In addition to completing the final HidroQoL version, data were also collected on other PROs such as the DLQI, the EQ-5D-5L, global impact question, time spent in managing the condition, patient demographic characteristics and disease characteristics/history.

Analysis

The distribution of the HidroQoL scores (items as well as scales) including mean, SD, maximum, minimum and frequencies for response categories (for the items) was estimated.

Correlation analysis, based on polychoric correlations, was carried out to identify items that were multicollinear. Correlation >0.08 indicates multicollinearity (Fayers and Machin 2007a, b).

Exploratory factor analysis (EFA) was carried out to explore the factorial structure of the HidroQoL. The optimal number of factors was determined by parallel analysis and confirmed using scree plots and goodness of fit statistics. Poorly performing items were identified based on highest loading below 0.4; more than one loading above 0.4, with none above 0.5; residual variance (uniqueness) of 0.7 or more; and content mismatch with their highest loading factor (Lackey et al. 2003; Costello and Osborne 2005; Nijsten et al. 2006) (see Chap. 2, Appendix, for the goodness of fit measures used).

T-test or its non-parametric equivalent such as Mann-Whitney was employed to assess known group validity. Spearman's correlation was carried out to assess convergence validity.

Findings

Score Distribution, Correlation Analysis and Factor Analysis

Criteria 1: responses should be evenly spread across response options, i.e. *the extreme ends (ceiling and floor) should not account for more than 15% of the sample.*

In total, 595 patients participated in the cross-sectional study.

For all items there was no response category accounting for more than 80% of responses, showing reasonable variability. Nevertheless, the items showed a negative skew reflecting some ceiling effects. In 44 items the highest response category 'very much' was chosen by 20% of participants. The ceiling effects were worse in 17 items where 50% of participants chose 'very much'. Items 'My choice of clothing is affected' (Q1), 'I feel embarrassed' (Q21), 'I feel self-conscious' (Q31) and 'I worry about people's reactions' (Q35) showed excessively large kurtosis. Thus the data shows some minor departure from normality. Nine items showed very low use (below 5%) of the lowest response category, 'no, not at all', and this includes 'My choice of clothing is affected' (Q1), 'My summer activities are affected' (Q10), 'I feel embarrassed' (Q21), 'I feel depressed' (Q25), 'My self-confidence is affected' (Q27), 'My outdoor activities are affected' (Q9), 'I feel self-conscious' (Q31), 'I worry about people's reactions' (Q35) and 'My whole life is affected' (Q49). This raises questions related to the utility of this category for these items. Missing data occurred at random and, for the items affected (Q18–Q49), was not more than 2% of responses. The incidence of missing data increased with successive items, starting from item Q18, reflecting drop-outs, as people who started responding to the questionnaire but stopped along the way. Withstanding the ceiling effects and the underuse of response category 'no, not at all', the distribution of responses was encouraging.

Various conclusions may be drawn from these findings. Most item scores show good variability with all options used, suggesting that the current response categorisation is relevant and is capable of discriminating among levels of HRQoL impairment. The ceiling effects observed in nearly all the items suggest that the current sample was experiencing severe HRQoL impairment or it may hint that the new PRO measure was not optimised for assessing an extreme level of impact. In which case, it may be necessary to reword the items to expand the bandwidth of severity in which the PRO measure may be used. Second, this may suggest that the specific validation sample includes patients with extreme levels of impact. Further investigation by looking at other distribution characteristics of the measure's scores may be necessary.

Criteria 2: individual items in a scale should not have a moderate to strong correlation, i.e. *rho > 0.08 indicates multicollinearity* (Fayers and Machin 2007a, b).

Spearman's correlations among the 49 items ranged from −0.03 to 0.92; 30 item pairs had a correlation of 0.8 or greater reflecting multicollinearity issues. This included 'I feel embarrassed' (Q21) against 'I feel nervous' (Q22) and 'I feel self-conscious' (Q31); 'My self-confidence is affected' (Q27) against 'My self-esteem is affected' (Q28) and 'I feel self-conscious' (Q31); and 'I have difficulties holding objects' (Q4) against 'I have difficulties handling money' (Q5), 'I find it hard to touch other people' (Q6), 'I find it hard to handle paper' (Q13) and 'I have difficulties using touch technologies (e.g. computer keyboard, smartphones)' (Q16).

Therefore 'My outdoor activities are affected' (Q9) and 'My summer activities are affected' (Q10) were removed. In the case of the collinearity between item 'I have difficulties using touch technologies (e.g. computer keyboard, smartphones)' (Q16) and items 'I have difficulties holding objects' (Q4) and 'I find it hard to handle paper' (Q13), item Q16 was removed. This was based on its lesser prevalence during qualitative research (Chap. 3) and the narrower conceptual breadth. The item 'My whole life is affected' (Q49) was unique; as a general impact question, it reflected a general view of respondents' condition summing up all aspects already addressed by the rest of the items. This suggests that it was overlapping with the rest of the instrument's items. Therefore, item Q49 was also removed, despite showing no correlation above 0.8 with any of the remaining items. This stage led to a 36-item version of the developmental HidroQoL (HidroQoL-36). The final version of the HidoroQoL following the first item reduction contained 36 items.

Exploratory Factor Analysis (EFA) of the HidroQoL

Following correlation analysis, exploratory factor analysis was carried out on the HidroQoL to explore its dimensional structure as well as to perform item reduction. First, the optimal number of factors to be extracted was determined, and then the factors were estimated. The poorly performing items were dropped in subsequent iterations until a 'simple structure was achieved'. According to Thurstone's criteria, a simple structure is characterised by a few high loadings on each factor with the rest of the loadings being zero or close to zero with variables having significant multiple loadings being at a minimum (Kline 1994).

Three factors were firstly extracted from the EFA of the HidroQoL-36, based on Horn's parallel analysis criterion and supported by the scree-plot criterion. Three factors laid to the left side of the elbow on the plot; the rest of the factors from the fourth going to the right were rubble, with the fourth factor also marking a change in the slope of the curve. The Goodness of fit index criteria showed mixed results. Although the chi-square test of model fit was significant (chi-square = 2316.34, df = 525, $p = 0$) indicating poor fit of the three-factor solution, the practical fit indices suggested otherwise (RMSEA = 0.078, SRMR = 0.51, CFI = 0.934, TLI = 0.921).

A further step following EFA of the 36-item set involved removing items that showed poor performance, to enhance the structure of the instrument. By examining the relationship between the individual items and their related constructs, the best items could be identified and selected (Gorsuch 1997). Following 10 analyses of the factor pattern matrix, a revised 21 items remained.

Revised HidroQoL: 21-Item Set

Ultimately, the iterative item reduction process yielded a set of 21 items which fitted to a two-factor solution (Tables 6.1 and 6.2, Analysis 10). Six items loading onto the first factor were related to 'daily life activities', for example, 'My physical activities are affected' (Q8), 'My everyday housework is affected' (Q11) and 'I worry about the additional chores in dealing with my condition' (Q45). Fifteen items loaded onto the second factor, and these were related to psychosocial impact and included 'I worry about people's reactions' (Q35), 'I feel embarrassed' (Q21), 'I feel nervous' (Q22), 'I feel sad' (Q24), 'I avoid public speaking' (Q12) and 'I do not socialise as much as I would like to' (Q17). The two factors correlated strongly (rho = 0.645), suggesting that a single factor solution might fit the data. Moreover, Horn's parallel analysis and scree plot favoured a single factor solution. However, the two-factor solution showed much better fit based on goodness of fit statistics.

Item-test correlation ranged from 0.68 (Q44) to 0.78 (Q3), for the 'daily life activities impact' factor, and from 0.7 (Q12) to 0.83 (Q36) for the psychosocial impact domain. The coefficient alpha estimates were 0.83 and 0.94, for the daily activities and the psychosocial impact domain, respectively.

Table 6.1 Factor pattern matrix and residual variances for the 21 items of the HidroQoL

Item	Factor pattern					Factor structure	
	F1	SE	F2	SE	Res. Var	F1	F2
Q8	0.89	0.019	0.004	0.003	0.204	0.892	0.578
Q11	0.832	0.043	−0.144	0.053	0.441	0.74	0.393
Q7	0.632	0.04	0.133	0.046	0.475	0.718	0.541
Q45	0.593	0.052	0.235	0.061	0.414	0.744	0.618
Q3	0.563	0.037	0.292	0.042	0.385	0.752	0.655
Q44	0.529	0.051	0.215	0.059	0.527	0.668	0.556
Q29	0.176	0.048	0.645	0.041	0.406	0.592	0.759
Q15	0.168	0.048	0.578	0.044	0.513	0.541	0.686
Q30	0.129	0.04	0.756	0.034	0.286	0.616	0.839
Q12	0.082	0.052	0.66	0.045	0.489	0.507	0.712
Q20	0.079	0.042	0.729	0.035	0.388	0.55	0.78
Q26	0.027	0.051	0.782	0.04	0.362	0.531	0.799
Q37	0.015	0.045	0.773	0.037	0.387	0.513	0.783
Q24	0.011	0.04	0.838	0.032	0.285	0.552	0.845
Q21	0.004	0.046	0.864	0.034	0.249	0.561	0.866
Q36	0.001	0.03	0.87	0.024	0.242	0.562	0.871
Q17	0	0.033	0.867	0.026	0.248	0.56	0.867
Q27	−0.069	0.038	0.926	0.027	0.22	0.528	0.882
Q22	−0.083	0.041	0.898	0.029	0.283	0.497	0.845
Q18	−0.115	0.041	0.933	0.03	0.254	0.487	0.859
Q35	−0.171	0.049	0.935	0.034	0.303	0.432	0.825

Table 6.2 Steps during EFA analysis: removal of poorly performing items

Analysis	Poor-load	Cross-load	Res_var > 0.7	Factor# -K's rule	Factor# -Paral	Factor# extract	RMSEA	SRMR	CFI	TLI	Chi-1	Chi-2
1. All 36 items	Q33, Q14	Q42, Q32, Q47, Q34, Q48, Q7	–	6	3	3	0.078 (0.075, 0.081)$p = 0.000$	0.051	0.934	0.921	2316.34 df = 525 $p = 0$	27716.08 df = 630 $p = 0$
2. Remove Q33	Q14	Q42, Q32, Q47, Q34, Q48, Q7	Q1	6	3	3	0.079 (0.076, 0.083)$p = 0$	0.051	0.933	0.922	2233.99 df = 493 $p = 0$	27396.52595 $p = 0$
3. Remove Q14	–	Q42, Q32, Q47, Q34, Q48, Q7	Q1	5	3	3	0.078 (0.075, 0.082)$p = 0$	0.05	0.94	0.93	2039.42 df = 462 $p = 0$	26958.234 df = 561 $p = 0$
4. Remove Q32 and Q42	–	Q47, Q34, Q48, Q7	Q43, Q1	5	3	3	0.82 (0.078, 0.085)$p = 0$	0.05	0.942	0.928	1908.4 df = 403 $p = 0$	26319.9 df = 496 $p = 0$
5. Remove Q34	–	Q47, Q48, Q7	Q43, Q1	5	3	3	0.084 (0.08, 0.088)$p = 0$	0.05	0.942	0.929	1859.1 df = 375 $p = 0$	26230.1 df = 465 $p = 0$

(continued)

Table 6.2 (continued)

Analysis	Poor-load	Cross-load	Res_var > 0.7	Factor# -K's rule	Factor# -Paral	Factor# extract	RMSEA	SRMR	CFI	TLI	Chi-1	Chi-2
6. Remove Q47, Q48	–	Q38, Q7	Q43*, Q1	5	3	3	0.086 (0.082, 0.090) $p = 0$	0.049	0.945	0.931	1646.39 df = 322 $p = 0$	24607.0 df = 406 $p = 0$
7, Remove Q38, Q1		Q7	–	5	2	3	0.089 (0.085, 0.094) $p = 0$	0.48	0.948	0.933	1491.1 $p = 273$ $p = 0$	23804.98 df = 351 $p = 0$
8, Remove Q2, Q4, Q13		–	Q43, Q6	4	2	2	0.099 (0.094, 0.104) $p = 0$	0.059	0.937	0.924	1490.17 df = 229 $p = 0$	20221.98 df = 276 $p = 0$
9, Remove Q43, Q6	–	–	Q39 (=0.7)	4	1	2	0.102 (0.096, 0.107)$p = 0$	0.055	0.944	0.932	1273.01 df = 188 $p = 0$	19726.8 df = 231 $p = 0$
10, Remove Q39	–	–	–	3	1	2	0.106 (0.101, 0.112)$p = 0$	0.056	0.944	0.93	1239.92 df = 169 $p = 0$	19305.35 df = 210 $p = 0$

A total of 163 participants completed the HidroQoL questionnaire, out of 204 initially enrolled for the study, representing 80% completion rate. One hundred and twenty-seven patients (78%) were from the USA and 36 (22%) the UK. The mean HidroQoL total score was 25.64 (±6.95) for the USA and 26.96 (±7.52) for the UK sample. The range for the HidroQoL total score was 2–36, in the USA group, and 1–33, in the UK group. Pooled data will be used in the analysis.

Known Group Validity

Hypothesis 1: Patients with severe disease would report lower HidroQoL scores in comparison with patients with less severe disease.

A comparison of HidroQoL scores across patients with different levels of disease severity, according to the HDSS score, was carried out using the Kruskal-Wallis (KW) test. Patients were grouped according to their HDSS score (HDSS = 2 versus HDSS = 3 or 4). Patients with HDSS = 1 were excluded from the study. The median overall and domain HidroQoL scores were statistically significantly higher in patients with HDSS = 3 or 4 in comparison with patients with HDSS = 2 ($p < 0.001$) (Table 6.3).

Hypothesis 2: Patients with disease involving more areas of the body would have lower HidroQoL scores.

The site of hyperhidrosis varied across patients in terms of location as well as number of sites, involving the following body regions—generalised, palms and feet, armpits, feet, palms and the head. HidroQoL scores of patients grouped according to site of hyperhidrosis were compared using the KW test. Two patient groups were created (generalised or ≥three areas of involvement versus ≤two sites). The median overall and domain HidroQoL scores were statistically significantly higher in patients with generalised or ≥three sites in comparison with the ≤two sites group ($p < 0.001$) (Table 6.3).

Table 6.3 Known group validity: comparison of median HidroQoL scores across patient groups according to skin area of involvement and disease severity (HDSS scores)

	Area of involvement			HDSS score		
HidroQoL scores, median [IQR]	≤two sites	Generalised or ≥ three sites	*P*-value (KW test)	1 or 2	3 or 4	*P*-value (KW test)
	$n = 111$	$n = 149$		$n = 51$	$n = 209$	
Total	27 [21.00, 31.00]	30 [24.00, 33.00]	0.002	21 [17.00, 24.50]	30 [25.00, 33.00]	<0.001
Daily life activities	9 [7.00, 11.00]	10 [8.00, 12.00]	0.023	8 [6.00, 9.00]	10 [8.00, 12.00]	<0.001
Psychosocial	18 [14.00, 20.00]	19 [16.00, 22.00]	0.003	14 [11.00, 17.00]	19 [17.00, 22.00]	<0.001

Convergence Validity

Hypothesis 1: The HidroQoL score is positively correlated with patient's HDSS score.

Testing this hypothesis involved assessing the degree and direction of association between the HDSS score and the HidroQoL's overall and domain scores. Spearman's rank sum correlation analyses were performed between the two measures. The coefficient of the Spearman's rank sum correlation showed significant association between the HDSS score and the HidroQoL overall and domain scores (total score rho = 0.58; daily score rho = 0.53, social score rho = 0.53) (Table 6.4). The focus of the HDSS on both severity and on interference in daily life activities places it closer to the content of the daily life activities domain than the psychosocial domain, explaining the small difference in the magnitude of the correlations.

Condition-specific QoL instruments given their attention on issues peculiar to a particular disease condition tend to have a greater connection to clinical outcomes. In this study, the HidroQoL has demonstrated a strong association with a standard clinical measure in hyperhidrosis, the HDSS. Moreover, it is noteworthy that the strong correlation has been achieved despite the absence of items related to 'symptoms' in the HidroQoL, highlighting the strong relevance of the items as a reflection of impacts arising from the symptoms of hyperhidrosis. Not only is the initial set of hypotheses confirmed, but these findings also give some preliminary indications on the capabilities of the instrument to detect change in patients over time.

Hypothesis 2: Patient's HidroQoL score was positively correlated with the DLQI score.

This hypothesis was assessed by estimating the Spearman's rank sum correlation between the HidroQoL scores and the DLQI total score. The HidroQoL scores showed moderate and positive correlation with the DLQI total scores (total score rho = 0.58; daily score rho = 0.51; social life rho = 0.54). This confirms our expectations that hyperhidrosis-specific QoL would be conceptually related to skin-specific QoL.

Hypothesis 3: The HidroQoL scores are not correlated with EQ-5Ds 'mobility' and 'self-care' domain scores.

Spearman's rank sum correlation analysis was used to assess the relationship between the HidroQoL scores and EQ-5Ds 'mobility' and 'self-care' domain scores. The scores for EQ-5Ds 'mobility' and 'self-care' domains showed no correlation with the HidroQoL scores ($p > 0.05$ in all instances). Similarly, the EQ-5Ds self-care domain score did not correlate with any of the HidroQoL scores, the total as well as the domain scores (Table 6.4). Our hypothesis is therefore confirmed, supporting the divergence validity of the HidroQoL, as the EQ-5D 'mobility' and 'self-care' domains deal with themes that are unrelated to the impacts of hyperhidrosis.

Table 6.4 Convergence validity: Spearman's rank sum correlation of the HidroQoL scores with other measures of disease burden

	A	B	C	D	E	F	G	H	I	J	K
HidroQoL total (A)											
HidroQoL daily (B)	0.84^{***}										
HidroQoL social (C)	0.95^{***}	0.64^{***}									
Time in managing hyperhidrosis (D)	0.20^{**}	0.24^{***}	0.16^{*}								
HDSS score	0.58^{***}	0.53^{***}	0.53^{***}	0.22^{***}							
DLQI score	0.58^{***}	0.51^{***}	0.54^{***}	0.20^{**}	0.41^{***}						
EQ5D5L_index	-0.33^{***}	-0.33^{***}	-0.28^{***}	-0.23^{***}	-0.32^{***}	-0.50^{***}					
MOBILITY	0.13^{*}	0.15^{*}	0.09	0.05	0.15^{*}	0.29^{***}	-0.69^{***}				
SELF_CARE	0.05	0.1	0.01	0.04	0.03	0.13^{*}	-0.46^{***}	0.39^{***}			
USUAL ACTIVITIES	0.29^{***}	0.30^{***}	0.25^{***}	0.14^{*}	0.29^{***}	0.41^{***}	-0.71^{***}	0.52^{***}	0.29^{***}		
PAIN_DISCOMFORT	0.20^{**}	0.23^{***}	0.16^{*}	0.22^{***}	0.20^{***}	0.34^{***}	-0.77^{***}	0.51^{***}	0.34^{***}	0.52^{***}	
ANXIETY & DEPRESSION	0.41^{***}	0.33^{***}	0.39^{***}	0.19^{**}	0.32^{***}	0.45^{***}	-0.68^{***}	0.29^{***}	0.12	0.37^{***}	0.32^{***}

Note: *P*-values of correlation coefficient: $^{***}p < 0.001$; $^{**}p < 0.01$; $^{*}p < 0.05$.

Hypothesis 4: The HidroQoL scores are correlated with EQ-5D-5L domains on 'usual activities', 'anxiety/depression' and 'pain or discomfort'.

Spearman's rank sum correlation analysis was used to assess the relationship between the HidroQoL scores and the EQ-5D-5L 'usual activities', 'anxiety/depression' and 'pain or discomfort' domains. The EQ-5D-5L score for 'usual activities' domain correlated with the HidroQoL scores (overall score rho = 0.278; daily life score rho = 0.299; psychosocial score rho = 0.230, $p < 0.01$). Slightly larger and significant correlations were also observed between the EQ-5D-5L 'anxiety/depression' domain scores and HidroQoL scores (total score rho = 0.387; impact on daily life activities rho = 0.339; psychosocial score rho = 0.363). Equally, the 'pain/discomfort' EQ-5D domain score correlated with the HidroQoL scores (total score rho = 0.254; daily life score rho = 0.271; psychosocial score rho = 0.215). This confirms our set hypothesis and demonstrates the similarities between hyperhidrosis-QoL and the mentioned domains of the EQ-5D-5L.

Hypothesis 5: Greater impairment in quality of life is associated with more time spent in managing the condition.

The relationship between HidroQoL scores and the daily time spent in managing the condition (measured in minutes) was assessed using Spearman's rank correlation analysis. The HidroQoL score showed moderate correlation with daily management time (overall scale score rho = 0.474; daily life score rho = 0.569; and psychosocial domain score rho = 0.372). This is consistent with our expectations and supports the notion that living with a long-term condition usually involves patients regularly taking treatment to address either symptoms or impacts of their condition, in addition to other measures to adapt to their condition. Both of these may be time consuming and may be associated with some QoL impairment.

Part II: Assessing How Well a PRO Measure can Be Used without Errors—Reliability

The centrality of HRQoL as the ultimate measure of disease impact and efficacy of drug therapies is clear. The current challenge, however, is in how to transform the process of measuring, collecting and applying HRQoL within the clinic, from guesswork into science (Finlay 2011). This is particularly relevant in skin disease where the impairment in HRQoL is profound (Finlay 1998) and represents a key indicator of disease activity. Part of the task entails ensuring that measurement instruments produce valid and reliable results. The latter means that an instrument produces measurements that are free of measurement error (Fayers and Machin 2007a, b; Lohr 2002). In multi-item scales measuring unidimensional concepts, where items are assumed to be indicators of a single underlying construct, reliability is demonstrated in internal consistency. The degree to which the different items forming the scales are homogenous or whether they tap into different components of differing constructs (Fayers and Machin 2007a, b).

Reliability is central to the measurement process such that it has an impact on other attributes of an instrument. For example, poor reliability may obscure correlation of a measure with other measures, in the assessment of convergence validity. On the other hand, an instrument's ability to detect change over time, responsiveness, is equally affected by poor reliability. Fundamentally, reliability is not a property of an instrument, but only an indication of the degree of reliability related to the use of an instrument in specific target populations and in a specific setting (Streiner and Norman 2008). This means that reliability may vary with target population and application of an instrument, indicating the need for establishing reliability each time a measure is put to a new use.

Overall, internal consistency shows that the instrument is capable of identifying variability in patients' conditions (Streiner and Norman 2008) and that each of the included items contributes to measuring the underlying concept. Where an instrument is used across time, reliability can be demonstrated by intertemporal reproducibility of scores, i.e. during test-retest assessment. This reflects the degree to which an instrument yields stable scores over time, with repeated administration, among respondents whose status on the concept of interest is unchanged (Lohr 2002). This entails that test-retest reliability can only be determined in a longitudinal context and that it relies on the assumption that the patient's condition has indeed not changed.

Two forms of reliability were assessed:

- Internal consistency of the scores for the impact on daily life activities and psychosocial impact domains of the HidroQoL and the overall scale score
- Test-retest reliability of the individual items of the HidroQoL, the scores for the impact on daily life activities and psychosocial impact domains and the overall scale score

Methods

This study followed a prospective longitudinal study design with patients assessed on two occasions, at baseline (assessment 1) and follow-up (assessment 2) at least 7 days after initial assessment. This interval has been recommended as offering a good balance between avoiding 'learning effects' in the second assessment and 'ensuring that change in the construct being measured does not take place' (Salek and Luscombe 1992; Streiner and Norman 2008). In addition, even though patients may experience much variability in their sweating on a day-to-day basis, the overall impacts on their life are relatively stable over a number of days. Moreover, effects of hyperhidrosis treatments such as oral systemic drugs or iontophoresis last 5–14 days, during which time little change may be expected.

Apart from the HidroQoL questionnaire, patients were also asked to complete the HDSS, a validated single item scale for assessing the severity of sweating and its interference on patient's daily life (Kowalski et al. 2004). This instrument has been reviewed in Chap. 1. To assess reproducibility of the HidroQoL scores, the level of agreement between scores from the first (baseline) and second (follow-up) assessments was assessed using intraclass correlation (ICC).

Findings

Internal Consistency

Internal consistency of the HidroQoL was assessed for the UK and the US samples separately and for the pooled patient population combining patients from all countries, using the baseline and follow-up scores. In the pooled sample, the Cronbach's alpha estimates of the HidroQoL overall scale were 0.89 and 0.93, for test 1 and test 2, respectively (Table 6.5).

Coefficient estimates for the impact on daily life activities domain (H-DA) were 0.76 and 0.86; and for the psychosocial impact domain (H-PS), they were 0.86 and 0.90, for test 1 and test 2, respectively. Estimates obtained from the US sample were larger, while those from the UK sample were the smallest, although all within a percentage point margin of difference. Optimal homogeneity is reflected in moderate inter-item correlation and moderate-to-strong corrected item-total correlations (Streiner and Norman 2008). This was, therefore, also examined for each of the HidroQoL's items. In the pooled sample, corrected item-total correlation ranged from 0.376 to 0.618. The lowest correlation was seen on item 1 (My choice of clothing is affected, rs = 0.376), while that for item 15, rs = 0.618, was the highest. In the US sample, corrected item-total correlations ranged from 0.410 to 0.664. Item 'I feel frustrated' (item 9) had the highest correlation, while the lowest was seen on 'My sex life is affected' (item 18).

In the UK group, the values of item-total correlation ranged from 0.24 to 0.739. The item 'I avoid meeting new people' (item 15) had the highest item-correlation

Table 6.5 Internal consistency* of the HidroQoL: Cronbach's alpha

HidroQoL score	Pooled sample	
	Test 1	Test 2
Overall scale, 18 items	0.89	0.93
Impact on daily life activities	0.76	0.86
Psychosocial impact	0.86	0.90

Note: *Cronbach's alpha coefficient.

value, while the lowest value was seen on item 'My choice of clothing is affected' (item # 1). This indicates that the HidroQoL is well balanced, as no item carried too much weight; each of the included items tapped an aspect of the underlying construct (hyperhidrosis QoL), including the item 'My choice of clothing is affected'. On the other hand, the items 'I feel frustrated' and 'I avoid meeting new people' appeared to highlight the experiences of having hyperhidrosis, in summing up the emotional and social impacts of the disease experienced by the patient.

Inter-Temporal Stability of the HidroQoL Scores

The reproducibility of the HidroQoL scores in repeated administration was tested. Patients completed the HidroQoL on two occasions, at baseline (test 1) and follow-up assessment (test 2). A central issue in the reliability relates to ensuring that the patients' condition has not indeed changed. One approach is to use a reasonably short time frame, to ensure that the underlying condition of the patient does not change but not too short to risk the patients recalling the prior responses. In this study patients took the follow-up assessment 5–7 days after initial assessment. On the other hand, patients also completed the HDSS scale, a self-assessment disease severity scale. Test-retest reliability of the HidroQoL was assessed only in patients whose underlying disease severity had not changed.

A total of 144 patients (pooled population) completed the second assessment out of the 260 patients completing the initial assessment, 104 patients showed no change on their HDSS score between the first and second assessments, and therefore only these were considered in the analysis. The level of agreement between the baseline (test 1) and follow-up scores (test 2) was assessed using ICC. In the pooled sample, the level of agreement in the HidroQoL scores was strong (ICC: overall scale score, 0.92; H-DA, 0.8; H-PS, 0.91) (Table 6.6).

The individual item scores also showed a strong reproducibility (ICC range, 0.74 to 0.88). The ICC for item 5 (I worry about additional activities in dealing with my condition) was the lowest (ICC = 0.59). In the US sample, similar results were observed (ICC: overall scale scores, 0.92; H-DA, 0.89; H-PS, 0.90). The ICC of the individual item scores ranged from 0.654 to 0.88. Item 5 (I worry about the additional activities in dealing with my condition) showed the lowest ICC (0.456).

The UK patient population was small ($n = 22$); thus the obtained estimates may be considered as preliminary only. The HidroQoL showed strong test-retest reliability in the UK patient population. ICC was 0.93 for the total score, 0.87 for impact on daily life activities domain and 0.92 for the psychosocial impact domain. At the individual item level, ICC was lowest for the item 'I worry about the additional activities in dealing with my condition' (ICC = 0.59) and ranged from 0.65 to 0.93 for the rest of the items.

Table 6.6 Test-retest reliability for individual items of the HidroQoL, pooled sample ($n = 104$)

			95% CI		
		ICC	Lower	Upper	Sig
1	My choice of clothing is affected	0.741	0.620	0.824	0.0001
2	My physical activities are affected	0.799	0.704	0.863	0.0001
3	My hobbies are affected	0.831	0.747	0.886	0.0001
4	My work is affected	0.740	0.619	0.823	0.0001
5	I worry about the additional activities in dealing with my condition	0.592	0.402	0.722	0.0001
6	My holidays are affected (e.g. planning, activities)	0.768	0.660	0.842	0.0001
7	I feel nervous	0.860	0.793	0.904	0.0001
8	I feel embarrassed	0.874	0.816	0.914	0.0001
9	I feel frustrated	0.760	0.648	0.836	0.0001
10	I feel uncomfortable physically expressing affection (e.g. hugging)	0.770	0.663	0.843	0.0001
11	I think about sweating	0.718	0.587	0.808	0.0001
12	I worry about my future health	0.822	0.739	0.879	0.0001
13	I worry about people's reactions	0.741	0.610	0.826	0.0001
14	I worry about leaving sweat marks on things	0.779	0.673	0.850	0.0001
15	I avoid meeting new people	0.879	0.823	0.918	0.0001
16	I avoid public speaking (e.g. presentations)	0.798	0.702	0.863	0.0001
17	My appearance is affected	0.848	0.777	0.897	0.0001
18	My sex life is affected	0.876	0.814	0.916	0.0001
	HidroQoL—Daily life activities	0.883	0.828	0.921	0.0001
	HidroQoL—Psychosocial domain	0.914	0.868	0.943	0.0001
	HidroQoL total	0.926	0.885	0.952	0.0001

Part III: Evaluating Ability to Capture Changes in Patients' Condition—Responsiveness

Where an instrument is used in a longitudinal context, for example, for monitoring the condition of individual patients over time, further psychometric attributes apart from internal consistency, reliability and construct validity may be required to ensure valid measurements. The measure must be capable of detecting important changes taking place in the patient's condition even if they are small, an attribute referred to as responsiveness (Guyatt et al. 1987). The assessment of responsiveness requires an external measure as a criterion for determining whether the patient's condition has changed, improved or worsened (Revicki et al. 2008). Previous clinical trial results, on differences between placebo and active treatment, or known distribution properties of the target patient population may also be useful as basis for assessing responsiveness.

Establishing responsiveness requires demonstrating that the observed score changes reflect true changes in the concept being measured (longitudinal validity) and that such changes are not merely random variability (longitudinal reliability) (Terwee et al. 2003). Moreover, as measurement error increases, a larger and larger magnitude of change might be required to demonstrate any treatment effect (Guyatt et al. 1987), reflecting an inverse relationship between reliability and responsiveness, similar to the observation on construct validity.

Methods

The focus of these analyses was to assess:

- Whether the HidroQoL was sensitive to change in patients whose condition had changed
- Whether the HidroQoL was capable of discriminating between patients experiencing different levels of change in their sweating

The patient population used in the assessment of construct validity and reliability was employed. This study followed a prospective longitudinal study design with patients assessed on two occasions, at baseline (assessment 1) and during a follow-up assessment (assessment 2) at least 21 days after initial assessment. There is no recommendation regarding the best interval between assessments in responsiveness studies. However, groups of patients expected to change should be identified a priori as is the case in other construct validation procedures.

In addition to the HidroQoL, data were also collected on the HDSS, the DLQI and patient demographic characteristics. Change in HidroQoL scores over 21 days was assessed using paired *t*-test. In addition, Cohen's effect size and standard response mean were also estimated.

Findings

The mean HidroQoL scores were 26.64 (±7.14) and 25.08 (±8.38), for baseline (test 1) and follow-up (test 2) assessments, respectively, and the range was 1–36 for both assessments. The mode scores were 33 (test 1) and 32 (test 2), suggesting high levels of QoL impairment in both assessments. The DLQI mean scores were 10.13 (±6.87) and 9.55 (±6.96), during the first and second assessment, with ranges of 0 to 25 and 0 to 26, respectively. This reflects moderate to very large life impacts; the lower cut-off for very large effect QoL effect for the DLQI is 11 (Hongbo et al. 2005a, b). Most patients had low to moderate scores, as reflected in the interquartile range (5–16) and (4–15) for both the first and second assessment, respectively, with no patients towards the upper extremity. The DLQI scores showed a slightly positive skew.

Patients were grouped according to the change in the HidroQoL between the two assessments, as follows: based on HDSS change score. Three groups were formed, patients not experiencing any change (HDSS change score = 0), patients who worsened (HDSS change score = 1) and patients who improved (HDSS change score = −1).

A paired *t*-test was carried out to assess the HidroQoL's sensitivity to change in each of the three patient groups: no change, worsened and improved. Patients in the improving group showed significant change in their HidroQoL-PS domain score ($p < 0.01$) and the total HidroQoL score ($p < 0.01$) (Table 6.7). The HidroQoL-DA domain score showed no significant changes in this group ($p = 0.08$). On the other hand, patients in the worsening group did not change in a significant way ($p > 0.05$) in their total and domain HidroQoL scores. The magnitude of the mean change scores between the improving and the worsening groups were comparable (mean score change, 3.1 ± 3.9 and −3.0 ± 5.3, respectively) indicating some asymmetry. However, the 'no-change' group still showed unexpected change. Results on Cohen's ES and standard response mean are reported in Appendix.

In longitudinal HRQoL measurement, it is important for an instrument to be capable of discriminating between patients experiencing different levels of change over time (Stratford and Riddle 2005). A one-way ANOVA test of the change scores across patient groups showed significant differences on the overall score, and the psychosocial domain score (overall HidroQoL score, $p = 0.026$; psychosocial domain score, $p = 0.035$; impact on daily activities, $p = 0.05$) showed non-significant differences.

Part IV: Establishing Criteria for Interpreting Scores of Patient-Reported Outcomes

Establishing that an instrument produces reliable and valid measures and that it is responsive may not be sufficient to render it useful in routine clinical practice or in clinical research. Information facilitating assigning of easily understood meaning to an instrument's quantitative scores must also be available (Lohr 2002).

Table 6.7 Change in HidroQoL scores across patient groups

Patient group	Score	Mean	SD	SE mean	95% CI		t	df	*p*-value
					Lower	Upper			
No change ($n = 64$)	HidroQoL-DA	0.64	2.24	0.28	0.08	1.2	2.29	63	0.03
	HidroQoL-PS	0.94	2.96	0.37	0.2	1.68	2.53	63	0.01
	HidroQoL	1.58	4.49	0.56	0.46	2.7	2.82	63	0.01
Worsening group ($n = 6$)	HidroQoL-DA	−1.5	1.64	0.67	−3.22	0.22	−2.24	5	0.08
	HidroQoL-PS	−1.5	3.83	1.57	−5.52	2.52	−0.96	5	0.38
	HidroQoL	−3	5.25	2.14	−2.51	8.51	1.4	5	0.22
Improving group ($n = 20$)	HidroQoL-DA	1.05	2.44	0.55	−0.09	2.19	1.93	19	0.07
	HidroQoL-PS	2.05	2.48	0.55	0.89	3.21	3.7	19	0
	HidroQoL	3.1	3.85	0.86	1.3	4.9	3.6	19	0

Note: HidroQoL-DA is HidroQoL daily activities domain, HidroQoL-PS is HidroQoL psychosocial impact domain

Rather than just knowing whether patient scores have changed in a statistically significant way, of relevance to patient management is whether a change in scores is clinically significant, i.e. whether the change in scores is large enough to have an implication for patient care (Wyrwich et al. 2005). Such a cut-off change score is considered as the minimum clinically important difference (MCID) (Guyatt et al. 2002). Also, for a given absolute score, clinicians may want to know its implication on the patients' condition, whether it represents a mild, moderate or severe state of the patient's condition. In widely used dermatology QoL instrument such as the DLQI, both score categorisation and qualitative descriptors for each band have been provided (Hongbo et al. 2005a, b; Prinsen et al. 2009). In addition, values for minimum clinically important difference (MCID) have been reported (Both et al. 2007; Basra et al. 2008). Nevertheless, efforts to ensure that QoL scores are interpretable are not limited to the above, and results of clinical trials and statistical characteristics of samples where the measure was previously used and comparative data from non-diseased populations may be useful. Availability of any of such data is therefore considered among the important psychometric attributes of an instrument.

Methods

To estimate the minimal clinically important difference (MCID) for the HidroQoL scores using anchor-based and distribution-based methods.

The estimation of the MID based on the anchor approach involved first grouping patients according to their HDSS-cs, score of −1, as slightly improved; score of 0, as experiencing no change; and score of 1, as slightly deteriorating. The mean score change in the slightly improving group provides the MID estimate (Crosby et al. 2003).

The MID for the HidroQoL was also estimated by integrating the anchor-based and distribution-based methods, i.e. using statistical characteristics of patient groups defined based on the external anchor. The upper bound for 95% CI of the mean HidroQoL-cs of the group that had not changed was estimated as a measure of MCID (de Vet et al. 2007).

A third approach used in establishing cut-offs for important change utilised the statistical characteristics of the sample of baseline patient responses ($N = 64$). Specifically, the standard deviation (1/2 SD and 1/3 SD) and standard error of measurement were estimated.

Findings

Anchor-Based Approach

Over the 21-day follow-up period, 71 percent of the patients ($N = 64$) registered no change in their condition on the HDSS (i.e. HDSS-cs = 0) (Appendix, Tables 6.11 and 6.12). No patient reported a major improvement/deterioration (i.e. HDSS-cs > 2). .

External measures (anchors) applied in assessing the clinical change in the patient's condition need to be easy to understand and intuitive to interpret and must correlate with the target scale as basis for confidence that they measure the target construct (Guyatt et al. 2002). The HDSS change score (HDSS-cs) had a correlation of −0.244 ($p = 0.021$) with the HidroQoL change score (HidroQoL-cs) (Table 6.8).

Integrated Approach

Using the integrated approach, MCID was estimated at 2.5, based on patients whose condition had not changed (i.e. HDSS change = 0) over 21 days; this was slightly higher for localised hyperhidrosis (~ 2.94) (Table 6.9).

Distribution-Based Approach

Using HidroQoL scores at baseline (i.e. day 1), the standard error of measurement (SEM) was 2.14, while the ½ SD was 3.39.

Table 6.8 Mean HidroQoL score change in the 'slightly improving' patient group as an estimate of the MCID

Site affected	Sample	*N*	Mean (day 1–day 21)	SD mean	SE mean	95% CI of mean	
All types	Pooled	19	2.84	3.78	0.87	1.02	4.66
	US	13	3.08	4.01	1.11	0.65	5.50
Localised	Pooled	16	2.63	3.67	0.92	0.67	4.58
	US	11	2.45	3.91	1.18	−0.17	5.08
Axillary	Pooled	14	2.93	4.08	1.09	0.57	5.29
	US	10	3.10	4.56	1.44	−0.16	6.36

Table 6.9 Upper bound of 1 tailed 95% CI for the mean HidroQoL change score in the 'no-change' patient group

Site affected	N	Mean (day 1–day 21)	SD mean	SE mean	Mean 95% CI		Mean + 1.645*SE
					Lower	Upper	1-tail, 95% CI
All types	64	1.58	4.49	0.56	0.46	2.70	2.50
Generalised	15	0.93	2.55	0.66	−0.48	2.34	2.02
Localised	49	1.78	4.93	0.70	0.36	3.19	2.94
Axillar	20	2.35	5.45	1.22	−0.20	4.90	4.36
Palmoplantar	45	1.38	3.99	0.59	0.18	2.58	2.36

Concluding Remarks

A single bespoke test of validity of PRO measures does not exist. The assessment of whether a PRO measure is fit for purpose and whether it measures what it purports to measure involves gathering different types of empirical evidence and testing various types of hypothesis. In this chapter, we have shown the different hypothesis tests and study designs that may be utilised to assess the psychometric properties of a new PRO measure. Specifically, the development of a measurement model and item reduction were performed in a large cross-sectional study. Psychometric testing of the final measure was carried in a longitudinal study with a 21-day follow-up. In general, findings of the two studies support the use of the new PRO (the HidroQoL) as a valid measure of disease-specific HRQoL impairment in hyperhidrosis.

Using correlation analysis and EFA, 28 items were removed from the measure, from an initial 49 items. Further, the results of the EFA identified 21 optimal items; these fitted to two domains interpretable as daily life activities impact and psychosocial domains. The single domain solution also showed good fit to the data.

Scales of the HidroQoL demonstrated strong internal consistency as well as intertemporal stability over a 7-day period. This means that each of the scales has been optimally defined and that each of the items indeed reflects a different aspect of the same core construct. In addition, where the HidroQoL is used longitudinally, score changes may be observed with minimal measurement noise.

Capability to discriminate across different levels of disease severity/size of area of involvement demonstrated by the HidroQoL is an important early indication of the ability to detect important changes in patients' condition (Fayers and Machin 2007a, b). Taken together this suggests that the HidroQoL would be useful in the clinic, for the diagnosis as well as management of hyperhidrosis.

The HidroQoL demonstrated expected moderate-strong correlations with other PROs/parameters of disease burden such as the DLQI score, HDSS score and time spent in managing hyperhidrosis. This supports our initial hypotheses and is consistent with what is known about hyperhidrosis—disease severity is based on interference in daily life, and disease-specific HRQoL is closely related to skin-specific HRQoL and some aspects of generic HRQoL. On the other hand, the lack of correlation between the HidroQoL score and EQ-5D-5L 'mobility' and 'self-care' domain scores is in line with expectation; hyperhidrosis is not known to have any impacts on mobility and self-care.

The HidroQoL demonstrated an ability to detect change; observed score changes over a 21-day follow-up period in the group with minimal improvement on the anchor parameter (i.e. HDSS score change of 1) were greater than in those who experienced no change (i.e. HDSS score change of 0). Score change in those improving (HDSS score change of +1) mirrored those whose condition worsened (HDSS score change of −1).

Information about what scores of a PRO measure actually mean in clinical terms, i.e. what a given score change actually means, is essential to the use of PRO information in decision-making in routine clinical practice as well as clinical research. Using anchor-based approaches as well as distribution-based approaches, the MCID estimates for the HidroQoL were estimated at 2.02–4.33, based on this an MCID of 2–3 as the most appropriate. The criteria used in the anchor approach—a score change of 1 on the HDSS has intuitive interpretation—map to a 50% change in the amount of sweating (Solish et al. 2007). On the other hand, the estimates based on distribution-based approach provide an estimate of the minimal detectable change, reflecting the precision of the new measure.

Appendix

Sample Size Considerations

Rules of thumb on sample size requirements for correlation analysis and factor analysis vary in their guidance, ranging from 5 to 20 observations per variable with more suggestions above and below this ratio (Costello and Osborne 2005). However, the minimum sample size required for accurate recovery of population factor pattern matrix is influenced by many factors including the distribution and reliability of the variables, degree of association among variables, communalities and degree to which factors are overidentified (Reise et al. 2000; Schmitt 2011). Thus power and precision ought to be core consideration in parametric estimation-based factor methods (Schmitt 2011), while in non-parametric approaches when communalities are high, sample size of 100 may be adequate (Reise et al. 2000).

Evaluating the Psychometric Properties of the HidroQoL

Table 6.10 Multicollinear items (correlations of at least 0.8)

Item	Related item
My choice of footwear is affected (Q2)	I feel uncomfortable in my shoes (Q40) I have problems with being barefoot (Q41)
I have difficulties holding objects (Q4)	I have difficulties handling money (Q5) I find it hard to touch other people (Q6) I find it hard to handle paper (Q13) I have difficulties using touch technologies (e.g. computer keyboard, smart phones) (Q16)
I have difficulties handling money (Q5)	I find it hard to touch other people (Q6) I find it hard to handle paper (Q13) I have difficulties using touch technologies (e.g. computer keyboard, smart phones) (Q16)
I find it hard to touch other people (Q6)	I find it hard to handle paper (Q13) I have difficulties using touch technologies (e.g. computer keyboard, smart phones) (Q16)
My physical activities are affected (Q8)	My outdoor activities are affected (Q9) My summer activities are affected (Q10)
My outdoor activities are affected (Q9)	My summer activities are affected (Q10)
I find it hard to handle paper (Q13)	I have difficulties using touch technologies (e.g. computer keyboard, smart phones) (Q16) I have problems with being barefooted (Q41)
I have difficulties using touch technologies (e.g. computer keyboard, smart phones) (Q16)	I have problems with being barefooted (Q41)
I do not socialise as much as I would like to (Q17)	I avoid meeting new people (Q18) I avoid going out (Q19)
I avoid meeting new people (Q18)	I avoid going out (Q19)
I feel embarrassed (Q21)	I feel nervous (Q22) I feel self-conscious (Q31)
I feel hopeless (Q23)	I feel sad (Q24) I feel depressed (Q25)
I feel sad (Q24)	I feel depressed (Q25)
My self-confidence is affected (Q27)	My self-esteem is affected (Q28) I feel self-conscious (Q31)
My self-esteem is affected (Q28)	I feel self-conscious (Q31)
I feel uncomfortable in my shoes (Q40)	I have problems with being barefooted (Q41)
I worry about the additional chores in dealing with my condition (Q45)	I worry about the additional time spent in dealing with my condition (Q46)

Table 6.11 Distribution of the HDSS score at baseline and 21 days

	Pooled sample	
HDSS score	Baseline (day 1)	Follow-up (day 21)
2	19 (21.3%)	27 (30.3%)
3	41 (46.1%)	38 (42.7%)
4	29 (32.6%)	24 (27%)

Table 6.12 Distribution of the anchors: HDSS change score and PGA score at 21 days follow-up

Anchor	Score	Number of patients
HDSS score Change	−1	19 (21.3%)
	0	64 (71.1%)
	1	6 (6.7%)

Table 6.13 Cohen's effect size and standard response mean of the HidroQoL change scores [day 0–day 21]

Patient group	HidroQoL scores	Test 1–Test 2		SRM			ES		
		Mean	SD	Est.	95% CI		Est.	95% CI	
					Lower	Upper		Lower	Upper
No change	Daily life activities	0.64	2.24	0.29	0.04	0.54	0.22	0.03	0.42
	Psychosocial	0.94	2.96	0.32	0.07	0.57	0.18	0.04	0.33
	Total	1.58	4.49	0.35	0.1	0.6	0.21	0.06	0.36
Minimally worsening	Daily life activities	−1.5	1.64	−0.91	−1.96	0.14	−0.81	−1.73	0.12
	Psychosocial	−1.5	3.83	−0.39	−1.44	0.66	−0.41	−1.52	0.69
	Total	−3	5.25	−0.57	−1.62	0.48	−0.6	−1.71	0.51
Minimally improving	Daily life activities	1.05	2.44	0.43	−0.04	0.9	0.36	−0.03	0.76
	Psychosocial	2.05	2.48	0.83	0.36	1.29	0.48	0.21	0.76
	Total	3.1	3.85	0.8	0.34	1.27	0.47	0.2	0.75

References

Basra MKA, Fenech R, Gatt RM, Salek MS, Finlay AY (2008) The dermatology life quality index 1994–2007: a comprehensive review of validation data and clinical results. Br J Dermatol 159(5):997–1035. https://doi.org/10.1111/j.1365-2133.2008.08832.x

Both H, Essink-Bot M-L, Busschbach J, Nijsten T (2007) Critical review of generic and dermatology-specific health-related quality of life instruments. J Investig Dermatol 127(12):2726–2739

Costello AB, Osborne JW (2005) Best practices in exploratory factor analysis: four recommendations for getting the most from your analysis. Pract Assess Res Eval 10(7):1–9

Crosby RD, Kolotkin RL, Williams GR (2003) Defining clinically meaningful change in health-related quality of life. J Clin Epidemiol 56(5):395–407

Fayers PM, Machin D (2007a) Scores and measurements: validity, reliability, sensitivity. In: Quality of life. John Wiley & Sons, Ltd, Hoboken, pp 77–108. https://doi.org/10.1002/9780470024522.ch4

Fayers PM, Machin D (2007b) Quality of life: the assessment, analysis and interpretation of patient-reported outcomes, 2nd edn. John Wiley & Sons, West Sussex

Finlay AY (2011) Practice gaps. Dermatologists should better integrate quality-of-life measures to inform and improve clinical decision making: comment on 'the impact of pruritus on quality of life. Arch Dermatol 147(10):1157. https://doi.org/10.1001/archdermatol.2011.266

Finlay AY (1998) Quality of life assessments in dermatology. Semin Cutan Med Surg 17:291–296

Gorsuch RL (1997) Exploratory factor analysis: its role in item analysis. J Pers Assess 68(3):532–560

Guyatt G, Walter S, Norman G (1987) Measuring change over time: assessing the usefulness of evaluative instruments. J Chronic Dis 40(2):171–178

Guyatt GH, Osoba D, Wu AW, Wyrwich KW, Norman GR (2002) Methods to explain the clinical significance of health status measures. Mayo Clin Proc 77(4):371–383

Hongbo Y, Thomas CL, Harrison MA, Salek MS, Finlay AY (2005a) Translating the science of quality of life into practice: what do dermatology life quality index scores mean & quest. J Investig Dermatol 125(4):659–664

Hongbo Y, Thomas CL, Harrison MA, Sam Salek M, Finlay AY (2005b) Translating the science of quality of life into practice: what do dermatology life quality index scores mean? J Investig Dermatol 125(4):659–664

Kline P (1994) An easy guide to factor analysis. Taylor & Francis Group, London. http://books.google.co.uk/books?id=6PHzhLD-bSoC

Kowalski JW, Eadie N, Dagget S, Lai PN (2004) Validity and reliability of the hyperhidrosis disease severity scale (HDSS). J Am Acad Dermatol 50:A.198. http://linkinghub.elsevier.com/retrieve/pii/S0190962203035345?showall=true

Lackey NR, Sullivan JJ, Pett MA (2003) Making sense of factor analysis: the use of factor analysis for instrument development in health care research. SAGE Publications Ltd, London. http://books.google.co.uk/books?id=5Jyaa2LQWbQC

Lohr KN (2002) Assessing health status and quality-of-life instruments: attributes and review criteria. Qual Life Res 11(3):193–205. https://doi.org/10.1023/a:1015291021312

Messick S (1988) The once and future issues of validity: assessing the meaning and consequences of measurement. Test Validity 33:45

Nijsten T, Unaeze J, Stern R (2006) Refinement and reduction of the impact of psoriasis questionnaire: classical test theory vs. Rasch analysis. Br J Dermatol 154:692–700

Prinsen CAC, Lindeboom R, Sprangers MAG, Legierse CM, de Korte J (2009) Health-related quality of life assessment in dermatology: interpretation of Skindex-29 scores using patient-based anchors. J Investig Dermatol 130(5):1318–1322

Reise SP, Waller NG, Comrey AL (2000) Factor analysis and scale revision. Psychol Assess 12(3):287

Revicki D, Hays RD, Cella D, Sloan J (2008) Recommended methods for determining responsiveness and minimally important differences for Patient-reported outcomes. J Clin Epidemiol 61(2):102–109

Salek MS, Luscombe DK (1992) Health-related quality of life assessment: a review. J Drug Dev 5:137–137

Solish N, Bertucci V, Dansereau A, Hong HC, Lynde C, Lupin M, Smith KC, Storwick G (2007) A comprehensive approach to the recognition, diagnosis, and severity-based treatment of focal hyperhidrosis: recommendations of the Canadian hyperhidrosis advisory committee. Dermatol Surg 33(8):908–923. https://doi.org/10.1111/j.1524-4725.2007.33192.x

Schmitt TA (2011) Current methodological considerations in exploratory and confirmatory factor analysis. J Psychoeduc Assess 29(4):304–321

Stratford PW, Riddle DL (2005) Assessing sensitivity to change: choosing the appropriate change coefficient. Health Qual Life Outcomes 3:23. https://doi.org/10.1186/1477-7525-3-23

Streiner DL, Norman GR (2008) Health measurement Scales : a practical guide to their development and use. Oxford University Press, Oxford. http://books.google.co.uk/books?id=UbKijeRqndwC

Terwee CB, Dekker FW, Wiersinga WM, Prummel MF, Bossuyt PM (2003) On assessing responsiveness of health-related quality of life instruments: guidelines for instrument evaluation. Qual Life Res 12(4):349–362

Terwee CB, Bot SDM, De Boer MR, van der Windt DAWM, Knol DL, Dekker J, Bouter LM, De Vet HCW (2007) Quality criteria were proposed for measurement properties of health status questionnaires. J Clin Epidemiol 60(1):34–42

de Vet HC, Ostelo RW, Terwee CB, van der Roer N, Knol DL, Beckerman H, Boers M, Bouter LM (2007) Minimally important change determined by a visual method integrating an anchor-based and a distribution-based approach. Qual Life Res 16(1):131

Wyrwich KW, Bullinger M, Aaronson N, Hays RD, Patrick DL, Symonds T (2005) Estimating clinically significant differences in quality of life outcomes. Qual Life Res 14(2):285–295

Part III

Practical Considerations When Applying PRO Measures

7 Integrating PRO Assessment in Clinical Trials, Routine Clinical Practice and Medicines Development Programmes

It is futile to have the most optimised PRO measure developed if it is going to gather dust on the shelf without any use. Whether a PRO measure can be easily integrated into clinical research or clinical practice may depend on several issues—specific to the PRO measure, factors related to the context of use and the potential users. This chapter is intended to discuss the process, key considerations and pitfalls in the application of PRO measures across the different settings – clinical trials, routine clinical practice, medicines regulatory and HTA processes. We have included findings from some of our research, first, to illustrate integration of PROs in palliative care and chronic pain clinics, and second, perspectives of industry executives and regulators on PROs. We conclude the chapter, with some recommendations on enhancing the application of PRO assessments across different settings.

This chapter will be presented in three parts:

- Integrating PRO measurements in clinical research
- PRO measurement in routine clinical practice: issues and special considerations
- Key considerations when using PRO information in drug development programmes/regulatory pathways
- Current topics: the utility of PRO information in streamlining flexible regulatory and access pathways

Part I: Integrating PRO Measurements in Clinical Research

The Role of PRO Assessments in Clinical Research.

The integration of PROs in clinical trials (intended for drug registration or otherwise) is not particularly new and may be traced back to the 1970s/1980s to clinical trials in CNS (e.g. for pain and migraine). Nevertheless, the renewed interest in assessing PRO endpoints may be linked to recent focus on patient centricity within

P. Kamudoni et al., *Living with Chronic Disease: Measuring Important Patient-Reported Outcomes*, https://doi.org/10.1007/978-981-10-8414-0_7

healthcare as well as need for more rigorous and comprehensive evidence base on outcomes in resource allocation decisions and drug benefit-risk assessments.

Given the many different types of PROs that may be assessed—*HRQoL, functional status, disease symptoms, satisfaction* and *utilities* – there may be a case for including at least one PRO concept in *all* clinical trials, as a direct measure of patient benefit as well as in order to comprehensively capture the outcomes of treatment. Capturing PROs may be particularly important in disease areas where disease activity or outcomes of interest are difficult to observe or measure clinically without patient report, such as exacerbation of asthma and pain. In cancer and illnesses where treatment has minimal impact on the length of life, the HRQoL or functional status may be particularly important. Similarly, the heavy toxicity associated with most cancer pharmaceutical treatments (e.g. chemotherapy) means that it is important to capture how these negatively affect the patient, in the overall assessment of the effectiveness of such treatments (benefit-risk evaluation). PROs may provide a basis for expanding the current understanding on modern cancer drugs, such as immunotherapies, where the nature of long-term effects and side effects is not fully understood.

Under the auspices of various international societies and professional colleges such as the OMERACT in rheumatology and EADV in dermatology, there are ongoing initiatives to encourage consistency in outcome measurement in RCTs. For example, the OMERACT Filter 2.0 framework identifies core aspects 'termed areas' of relevance in rheumatology—death, life impact, resource use and pathophysiological manifestations (Boers et al. 2014). Almost all domains identified under 'life impact' (e.g. ICF domains: activity and participation, QoL, health status), and some under pathophysiological manifestations (e.g. ICF: body function and structure), require information that only the patient may provide, i.e. PROs. If anything, this seems to suggest that as a minimum multiple PROs may be needed to appropriately capture the different aspects of disease manifestation and impact to be measured.

Steps in Integrating PROs into Clinical Research

The assessment of PRO endpoints has the same requirements, and perhaps even more, as other clinical trial endpoints. In the trial design and planning stage, clear definition of PRO endpoint objectives and hypothesis as well as selection of appropriate PRO measures are necessary. In the implementation phase, practical issues relating to training of sites, PRO measure administration and quality assurance are considered. In the data management and analysis stage, appropriately dealing with issues of data QA, missing data and multiplicity of endpoints is an issue. In the reporting stage, applying relevant standards such as the CONSORT PRO reporting. Issues of relevance for each stage are discussed in turn.

Clinical Trial Design and Planning Stage

Initially, to develop a PRO endpoint strategy, the relevant PRO concepts (e.g. specific symptoms) for a target population ought to be identified, for example, using literature review or exploratory qualitative research. Appropriate PRO measures are then selected based on the objectives of the clinical trial, the content and psychometric attributes of the measure, suitability to the target population and feasibility in the intended setting of use (Fayers and Machin 2007). PRO aspects also ought to be included in the main study protocol in detail, including, for example, PRO-specific hypothesis; PRO endpoint specification, the timing of PRO assessments; selection of PROs and relevant measures; PRO data collection plans; a priori definition of intended analyses; and ethics issues such as PRO-specific consent information (Calvert et al. 2013b).

Trial Implementation and Practical Stage

Methodological as well as organisational decisions during study design play an important role in shaping the data collection. For example, while the timing of PRO assessments needs to reflect hypothesis regarding the timing of maximal effects of the treatment and might be event- or time-driven, these may be scheduled to coincide with planned clinic visits driven by other trial endpoints. The PRO measures may be administered through self-completion or interview delivery, paper-and-pencil delivery or electronic delivery. If data collection is being undertaken within clinical settings, it is thought that PRO measures should be administered prior to patients seeing their clinicians, to minimise bias in the responses.

The assessment of PRO endpoints in large multinational studies may present unique challenges in comparison with single or multicentre single-country RCTs, well summed up in a recent work by Gnanasakthy and colleagues (Gnanasakthy et al. 2013a). First, the differences across countries due to culture, socioeconomic settings and language may introduce unnecessary variation and potential biases in the data highlighting the need for cultural adaptation of PRO measures (see Box 7.1 for an overview of the process of translation and cultural adaptation of PRO measures). Second, as the number of countries where an RCT is rolled out increases, the amount of preparation required, for instance, supplying the relevant versions of the PRO measures, training of staff on PROs and managing the data process, substantially increase. In addition, the amount of resources and time required for integrating PROs in RCTs should not be underestimated. Expertise from various disciplines, such as outcomes research, biostatistics/epidemiology and clinical research, is required. The processes of PROM selection, planning and organisation of data capture and training for study coordinators and patients require careful planning and resources. Further, in addition to the research questions that RCTs are attempting to address, multinational RCTs may also be geared at a larger number of stakeholders (health authorities across different countries)—which may have different views, priorities and preferences on treatment effect and the particular role of PROMs.

Data Management and Analysis Stage

The data management systems and processes must facilitate adequate monitoring of the data collection process, e.g. aspects such as compliance. These should allow real-time identification of potential problems and issues, e.g. push notifications or regular reporting. Key steps and procedures involved in transforming the

Box 7.1 Key Steps in the Translation and Cultural Adaptation of PRO Measures

Inclusion of PROs as endpoints in multinational trials raises the need for translation and cultural adaption of measures from an original culture (or language). This may also be an issue for a single language used across multiple countries, for example, Portuguese spoken in Portugal and Brazil.

Good research practices on language translation and cultural adaptation published by ISPOR (Wild et al. 2005) have recommended the following steps:

1. Preparation—Writing of a description of the concepts in a PRO measure.
2. Forward translation—More than one translation of PRO measure from original/source language to target language is performed.
3. Reconciliation—Multiple forward translations are merged into one by a translation panel, an independent native speaker or an appointed investigator.
4. Back translation—The merged forward translation is translated back into original language, by a native speaker(s) of the original language. Any discrepancies between the back-translation and the original version are explored.
5. Harmonisation—The final translation version is generated; this typically involves comparison of various back-translations with the original measure at a harmonisation meeting.
6. Cognitive debriefing – The respondent understanding of the translated version of the PRO measure is assessed. Results are compared against original measure, and necessary revisions performed.
7. Proof reading—Final translated instrument is checked for errors (e.g. spelling diacritical, grammatical) at the proofing stage.
8. Final report—All decisions made throughout the translation process, e.g. justification for choice of certain words, are documented.
9. Although the above steps are appropriate for country-specific adaptations of a single language, several alternative approaches could be considered in this setting: Developing different same-language versions for each country, adapting a measure from original culture into a new country and developing a universal translation version ~ used across multiple countries (Wild et al. 2009).

raw data from the sites to the final datasets analysed should be traceable. Unlike other endpoints, PRO often comes with scoring instructions of varying complexity; how and when these are applied during the flow of data must be transparent.

To ensure credibility, analyses performed ought to follow the specification in the protocol and statistical analysis plan (SAP). Depending on the definition of the PRO endpoints, this may involve descriptive analysis such as mean scores/change score from baseline, proportion of responders based on score cut-offs and multivariate analyses, where techniques allowing for adjustment of baseline characteristics, e.g. PROM scores, and patient demographic characteristics, such as ANCOVA, are employed.

Further, PRO data have various nuances such as following non-normal distributions and multidimensionality, i.e. multiple domains and scales for a single concept, which should be carefully considered in the planning of analyses. For instance, the level of significance used in statistical analyses may need to be adjusted for multiplicity; several PRO endpoints are being concurrently assessed. Furthermore, analyses need to take into account the nature of missing data, for example, using appropriate data imputation method. The implications of the analysis decisions on the results should also be considered, through sensitivity analysis.

The time dependency in PRO data has often been neglected in analyses. Methods that consider this in the estimation of treatment effect should be considered, e.g. generalised estimating equations, hierarchical multilevel models and MANOVA.

Results Reporting Stage

The reporting of PRO results in clinical trials has been generally suboptimal (Calvert et al. 2013b). For example, a systematic review including 65 prostate cancer RCTs (Efficace et al. 2014) found various reporting deficiencies such as lack of hypothesis related to PROs (reported in 37% of RCTs only), method of PRO administration (reported in 23% of RCTs only) and documentation of statistical methods for addressing missing data (18% of RCTs). A PRO extension of the CONSORT checklist has recently been developed to harmonise and enhance the reporting of PRO results in clinical trials (Calvert et al. 2013a). The checklist identifies five items which must be reported in all RCTs reporting PRO results: (1) identifying PROs as primary or secondary outcome in the abstract, (2) description of the hypothesis related to PROs as well as relevant domains, (3) references or psychometric evidence related to validity and reliability of PRO measure, (4) description of methods for addressing missing data and (5) discussion of study limitations specific to PROs as well as generalizability of PRO results to various populations.

It is hoped that better reporting of PRO trial results may not only influence translation of clinical trial results into clinical practice but also broadly encourage better planning and execution of PRO trials, as well as the clinical validity of results (Calvert et al. 2013b).

Part II: PRO Measurement in Routine Clinical Practice – Issues and Considerations

The growing interest in routine assessment of PROs in clinical practice as a way of systematically capturing and applying the perspective of the patient in the care process is one of the key developments in the field. There is often a disparity between the concerns experienced and described by patients and the clinicians' ability to identify and focus such issues (Schor et al. 1995; Beckman and Frankel 1984; Calkins et al. 1991; Siminoff et al. 1989). The feedback of information captured from PROMs to healthcare professionals is expected to facilitate patient-clinician communication, uncovering patients' problems and monitoring response to treatment (Higginson and Carr 2001). A growing number of studies support the feasibility of individual PRO reports using standardised measures and suggest that the majority of patients are willing to complete questionnaires as a routine part of their clinic visits (Detmar and Aaronson 1998; Cohen et al. 1997; Koller et al. 2005). A growing body of evidence demonstrates an increase in doctor-patient communication on HRQoL issues within the consultation following the feedback of PROM scores to clinicians (Velikova et al. 2004; Detmar et al. 2002). However, the beneficial effects of routine PRO assessment on the management of the patient or outcomes of patient care are still inconclusive (Valderas et al. 2005; Greenhalgh et al. 2005). Successful integration of PRO assessments into routine practice involves multiple steps and requires addressing various core issues. This section describes 'configuration and design of PRO assessment in the clinic' and 'issues and recommendations in assessing PROs routinely'.

Design and Configuration of Routine PRO Assessment

Design and configuration of PRO assessments is driven by the purpose for collecting PRO data, which indeed vary. The ISOQOL published a user guide on the topic 'User guide to Implementation of PRO Assessment in routine clinical practice', which has been summarised by Snyder and colleagues. Various useful articles on the topic are available.

Key steps in designing routine PRO assessments include:

1. Establishing the rationale for collecting PRO information involves:
   - Setting clear objectives for collecting PRO information, e.g. to support screening for specific symptoms or to enhance shared decision-making in the care process.
   - Defining the relevant target patient population providing the information, e.g. patients with psoriatic arthritis treated with a biologic. The target patient population's ability to provide reliable PRO information is an important consideration.
   - Identifying the target end-user of the PRO information such as nurse or doctor, based on the level of interest, willingness and ability to apply PRO information. These may vary across different specialties.
2. Identifying relevant PROs to be assessed and selecting appropriate measures:
   - The choice of PRO measures may depend on issues patients are most concerned about or aspects likely to be influenced by care provided (Snyder et al. 2014).
   - The risk here is to select a measure simply based on familiarity.

3. Defining a data collection strategy, encompassing both the setting in which questionnaires will be completed and the mode of administration and process of data collection:
   - PROMs may be completed 'at home' prior to healthcare visits or in the clinic prior or during consultation.
   - PROMs may be delivered as interviews or self-completion using paper-and-pencil versions, internet-delivered e-versions or computer device e-versions.
4. Establishing and defining criteria for supporting qualitative interpretation of PROM scores, e.g. for a questionnaire such as the Dermatology Life Quality Index (DLQI) what does a score of 18 out of a total score of 36 really mean? What would a 10-point score change represent?
5. Finding the most impactful way to report and present PRO information, bearing in mind the purpose of data collection and targeted end-user (please see Box 7.2 for suggestions on presentation of PRO information):
   - Patients and clinicians may have different preferences for presentation formats. In turn, different presentation formats vary in terms of perceived usefulness, ease of understanding and accuracy.
   - Line graphs tend to be preferred by both clinicians and patients (Brundage et al. 2015), with the representation of improvement using an upward trending line being the most accurately understood.
6. Developing decision aides with clear recommendations on actions to be taken based on PROM information. For example, PROM scores may be linked to prescribing of particular treatments or referral to specialist healthcare services.

Box 7.2 Impactful Presentation of PRO Data

The meaningful application of PRO data in routine clinical practice requires that PRO information or results are presented optimally in ways that facilitate accurate and easy understanding. The choice of types of graphics, formatting and labelling, has an influence on this. Several reports of empirical work assessing accuracy of interpretation and ease of understanding and usefulness of different formats of data presentation across different stakeholders, using mixed methods approaches, are now available (Brundage et al. 2015; Snyder et al. 2017).

Choice of graphics

- **For group-level data**, line graphs of means/medians with confidence intervals (CIs) have been ranked highest in terms of understanding and usefulness by both clinicians and patients (Snyder et al. 2017), in comparison to bubble plots or heat maps. *Bar graphs* were thought to be useful, by the clinicians, especially in making comparisons across treatment groups (e.g. average change or proportions corresponding to stable, worsening or improving groups). In contrast, *cumulative density function (CDF)* plots were found to be most difficult to interpret. Clinicians valued p-values, norms and confidence intervals, while patients found these confusing.

(continued)

Box 7.2 (continued)

- **For individual-level data**, most graphic formats were easily interpretable by clinicians. For *heat maps*, the colour coding was considered helpful, especially when simplified. *Tabular presentations* of scores while being clear were thought to present too much data and to be boring.

Directionality

- Depiction of improvement using an upward trending line, and worsening with a downward trending line, was considered intuitive and easy to interpret by both clinicians and patients.
- Thus, for example, for fatigue, where *higher scores = better* means, an upward trending line would represent lower fatigue, while *higher scores = more* means an upward trending line would represent higher fatigue.

Depicting clinical importance of scores

- Where scores are depicted as curves/trend lines, use of a 'threshold line' indicating normal versus concerning scores was found to be more easily and accurately understood than use of different shading or other ways of formatting line graphs.

Issues and Special Considerations

Assessment of PROs in clinical practice is intended to provide information applied in the management of the individual patient. Therefore, the processing, analysis and application of PRO information need to happen within the context of available time and resources within the clinic and in line with clinical flow. This presents unique issues for the patients completing the questionnaires and the healthcare professionals collecting and applying PRO information, PRO measures used and infrastructure supporting the process.

Patients

Quality of PRO information depends on patient's engagement with the assessments, with suggestions that the process of PROM completion may have a positive effect on patient well-being (Velikova et al. 2004). This is dependent on the relevance of a questionnaire's content to the patient, i.e. whether patients perceive these as representing their voice and experience. In addition, questionnaire completion should not require undue effort or on the patient. Disease-specific or individualised PROMs may have greater relevance for the patients in comparison to generic measures. The use of tailored measures through CAT administration offers an attractive option in the routine clinical practice setting for offering measures that are brief and related to severity of the concepts being assessed. Strategies for addressing various threats to data accuracy and quality should be put in place – addressing dynamics of the patient-doctor relationship, the context of assessments, the perception that responses provided may have an influence on ultimate care and other biases, i.e. 'social desirability bias'.

Clinicians

Inertia to change, for example, adoption of new clinical guidelines, is well known among clinicians. This is equally of concern for routine PRO measurement. This is associated with various factors including pessimism on the real benefit of structured PRO assessment in clinical practice, lack of knowledge and experience on PRO measurement, lack of information on interpretation of scores and lack of decision aides on applying PRO information.

Thus, planning and integration of PRO assessments should consider the training of all personnel involved to address any skills gaps and foster positive attitudes, fostering local ownership of PRO assessments process and targeting HCPs who would find PRO information most useful.

Resources and Infrastructure

Routine assessment of PROs in clinical practice requires resources and clear processes supporting data capture, analysis and ultimate application by end-users (i.e. target HCPs). This may require reconfiguration of existing clinical flow and processes, new IT infrastructure as well as appropriate training. Reimbursement of the time spent by HCPs in capturing and processing PRO information may be a strong incentive. For example, the inclusion of diabetes outcomes in the UK National Health Service Quality Outcomes Framework in 2004, whereby achievement of targets included in the framework influenced payment to GPs, was associated with a marked improvement in the quality and quantity of information on the outcomes included in the framework.

An Illustration of PRO Assessments in Clinical Practice

To illustrate the considerations and issues mentioned above, we discuss an example based on work carried out by our team to evaluate the practicality and value of routine HRQoL assessment in outpatient palliative care and chronic pain clinics over a 2-year period. Information from HRQoL assessments prior to consultation at every clinic visit was provided to clinicians (including a consultant psychiatrist, three specialist registrars in palliative medicine and a general practitioner clinical assistant). In the first year, the research team helped the clinical staff to manage and encode the HRQoL data and held regular meetings to improve implementation and assure that the staff were motivated. In the second year, the assessments continued but were run entirely by the clinic staff.

Implementation Process

Before each clinic, administrative staff attached the questionnaire to the medical records of all patients to be seen. On arrival, patients were registered and asked to complete the questionnaire in the waiting room before seeing the doctors.

Administrative staff and nurses were available to help with the questionnaire completion, if patients so wished. The completed questionnaires were returned to the receptionist and were then inserted in the front of the patient's medical record along with results of any investigations. These notes were then passed on to the clinic nurse, who arranged the consulting schedule, and finally to the doctors for the consultation. The doctors were asked to record which items of the patients' reported HRQoL they found helpful and the main interventions influenced by that information. All records were kept in the patients' medical file for future monitoring. The flow of information would have looked similar in an electronic-based system.

Health-Related Quality of Life Instrument

The McGill Quality of Life Questionnaire (MQOL) was selected for assessing HRQoL based on its practicality, relevance of content and evidence of reliability and validity in patients receiving palliative care (Cohen et al. 1997; Cohen and Mount 2000; Cohen et al. 2001). This measure contains 16 items, covering physical symptoms, physical well-being and psychological, existential and support domains, plus an overall quality of life assessment and an open-ended question on factors influencing the patient's quality of life. A previous study has demonstrated patient acceptability of the MQOL in routine clinical monitoring (Pratheepawanit et al. 1999). The revised format of the MQOL (R-MQOL), containing the two pages on one side of an A4 sheet, was used in this study to improve its practicality in clinical practice. The factorial structure and the psychometric properties of the R-MQOL were found to be acceptable and broadly consistent with the hypothesised structure of the original questionnaire.

Findings

A total of 1765 medical consultations took place during the 2 years, of which 1237 (70%) were evaluable. Five hundred and sixty patients attended the clinic during the study period. The average response from patients was 77% in the first and 64% in the second year. Palliative care accounted for 43% of consultations in the first year and 52% in the second year. No correlation was found between numbers of attending patients on a given day and the percentage of completed questionnaires. Completion of R-MQOL more than one time was 48% (range 1–22 times) in year 1 and 62% in year 2 (range 1–46 times over 2 years). Overall missing data on the R-MQOL was 2.22% in year 1 and 8.66% in year 2.

The response from the doctors regarding the use of the information from R-MQOL during consultations was very low (35% year 1; 12% year 2). Of 305 consultation records that included the doctor's view, the R-MQOL information had not helped clinical decision-making in only 10 (3%) consultations. More items were reported as useful in year 1 (mean 2.4; range 0–16) than in year 2 (mean 0.7; range 0–16) ($p < 0.001$). The doctors regarded physical symptoms (items 1 to 3, 55%) and the psychological domain (item 5, 58%; item 6, 50%) as the most useful.

Using year 1 data, 213 (33%) doctors' responses indicated which individual R-MQOL items were useful for specified interventions. Information on physical symptoms (68%) was useful when the doctors made interventions of changing medication, while psychological (62–68%) and existential (51–60%) domains were more useful when educating patients about their condition. A similar trend was reported in year 2.

Key Learnings from Case Study

1. The findings indicate that routine HRQoL assessment may be practical and beneficial in clinical practice. The implementation was run successfully by the clinical team over 2 years, although the response rate fell slightly during the second year when there was no support from the research group with data handling and maintaining motivation. The positive comments (97% of all comments from doctors) demonstrated the value of HRQoL information from the R-MQOL during consultations.
2. Taking into account the theory-driven approach suggested by Greenhalgh et al. (Greenhalgh et al. 2005), the positive results of HRQoL implementation in this study lie in many factors:
   (a) Firstly, the HRQoL measure used is a patient-centred approach with individualised items for physical symptoms, being completed on more than one occasion. As clinical decision-making is often a shared process in this setting, having HRQoL data available in a medical record for monitoring over time proved useful.
   (b) Secondly, regular meetings to solve barriers in implementation also promoted ownership of the measure for long-term use.
   (c) Thirdly and importantly, palliative care specialists and the psychiatrist and pain management clinician involving in the study acknowledged the value of HRQoL as the goal of their care. This was observed during regular meetings where physicians shared views about 'unrecognised' problems arising from the questionnaire and items that helped them get to the point that patients were distressed about and enabled the monitoring of their treatment. Routine information on emotional issues was useful, especially in complex cases where some patients 'put on a brave face'. Clearly, the data supported their comments, as the R-MQOL was used more frequently with patients who reported a poorer quality of life, suggesting that the doctors used such information more seriously when confronted with difficult cases.
   (d) Finally, with no interpretation or cut-off point of R-MQOL scores available, presentation of the whole questionnaire to the clinicians, just like other lab data, along with previous HRQoL scores (if any) for comparison was beneficial. It is suitable in this setting where the rating scale (range 0–10) is similar to pain scores that the clinicians are familiar with.

It should be noted that a minority of patients told their doctors at the time of consultation that the form was time-consuming and depressing, as it forced them to confront the reality of their feelings and symptoms. Although this study did not investigate this issue, it may well be a positive outcome. Some patients had perceived completion of additional R-MQOL questionnaires at follow-up visit as unnecessary duplication. This highlights the need to provide adequate information to patients on assessment of HRQoL in routine clinical practice.

The busy clinic might have played a part in the under-recording of the doctors' views. Sometimes the form was only partly completed when the patient was called in, so the doctors did not have the data at consultation. Doctors' motivation for the study varied, as clearly shown by a decrease in their response during the second year.

Overall, HRQoL self-assessment appears to quantify patients' experiences and therefore contribute to a more focused and effective doctor-patient interaction. The completion of the questionnaire itself may signal to patients that psychological aspects of their well-being are being recognised as important by the clinicians. Participation of patients in the process of care may also expand their sense of control over their illness, relieve anxiety and improve satisfaction (Wagner and Vickrey 1995; Detmar and Aaronson 1998). Thus, we feel that the benefits of routine HRQoL self-rating by patients exceed any burden that HRQoL measurement places on a minority of patients.

However, a response to a questionnaire will neither replace clinical interviews nor should be used as the sole measure of change in an individual without the support of biomedical evidence (Deyo and Carter 1992; Koller et al. 2005). When patient scores differ from clinicians' perceptions, the discrepancy can then be addressed by further in-depth discussion. The systematic HRQoL assessment can also enable doctors to monitor patients' condition over time and may encourage such information to be communicated effectively between professionals.

Although many doctors may have difficulty initiating such assessments, the notion forces a change in the culture of care towards a 'partnership culture' between patient and physician. Such a process requires involvement, education, training and ownership of the process, to ensure the success of HRQoL assessment in routine practice and the use of such information in clinical decision-making.

Part III: Applying PROs in Regulatory and Patient Access Pathways

Use of PROs in Market Authorisation Processes at the FDA and EMA

Interest in inclusion of PRO results in drug labels in recent years reflects the changing role of PROs within medicines authorisation procedures. Further, usefulness of PRO information goes beyond labelling claims, such as understanding of safety and efficacy evidence, e.g. experience of patients during progression-free survival. PRO labels were approved in 23% ($n = 70$ products) of all new molecular entities (NMEs) and biologic licence approvals (BLAs) at the FDA over the period 2000–2012 ($n = 308$) (Gnanasakthy et al. 2013a, b, c) and more frequently when used as a primary than as a secondary endpoint (Gnanasakthy et al. 2013a, b, c). There are notable differences in rates of PRO labels approved, across therapeutic areas. In CNS,

41% of all drug approvals from January 2006 to June 2012 included a PRO label (Gnanasakthy et al. 2013a, b, c). In contrast, the FDA oncology division carried out the largest number of reviews for PRO label claims in the period 2006–2010; however, no single PRO label was approved during this period (Hao 2010). A review of NMEs and BLAs evaluated by the OHOP during 2010–2014 showed that only 3 out of 40 drugs (24%) reviewed received a PRO label, while PRO information was included in the DAP of 13 drugs.

There is still misalignment across regulatory agencies such as the FDA and the EMA on their perception and use of PRO data. For example, PRO label claims granted at the FDA have primarily included disease-defining or proximal disease impact concepts, while generic or distal concepts such as quality of life and work productivity are less recognised. In contrast, the EMA has highlighted the importance of considering HRQoL, especially in disease areas such as oncology. For example, a review of five mCRPC drugs evaluated at the FDA and EMA revealed more PRO label claims granted by the EMA (n = 4, for pain, and n = 3, for HRQoL), than the FDA ($n = 2$, for pain) (Clark et al. 2014).

Despite numerous efforts to improve the quality of the PRO data submissions to regulatory agencies, there is still much room for improvement. Reviews of rejected PRO labelling claims in oncology (Hao 2010), and in other indications (DeMuro et al. 2013), at the FDA highlight several pitfalls, including:

- Inadequate fit for purpose: Weak evidence supporting the link between PRO concept assessed and labelling claim was considered weak.
- Study design weaknesses: Open-label designs were considered less credible due to biases related to the subjective nature of PROs. This was especially relevant in oncology and orphan diseases, where for ethical reasons, lack of sufficient population, RCTs are not feasible.
- Lack of information supporting the clinical meaningfulness of the PRO scores.
- Poorly planned and executed statistical analysis: the multidimensionality and multiplicity of PROs not adequately addressed, lack of a priori criteria for defining success or failure on PRO endpoint and lack of plans for addressing missing data.
- Lack of support for the administration of the PRO measure: lack of appropriate information to facilitate administration of the instrument, e.g. clear instructions and appropriate training.
- Ambiguity relating to treatment effect: change seen in only a single dimension or observed changes across dimensions/domains went in different directions.

Perspectives from Industry Executives and Regulators

To gain further insights on role and challenges related to use of PROs in regulatory processes and identify opportunities for mainstreaming this, our research team recently interviewed seven experts covering three different medicines regulatory agencies, regulatory affairs departments of three different large pharmaceutical companies and a global contract research organisation (CRO) that also deals with market access issues. All experts had more than 10 years of experience in the field and were senior in their organisations. The focus of the interviews was on the role of PROs in medicines regulation, to understand current issues and to explore opportunities for addressing these.

Common PRO-Related Issues Encountered in Regulatory Processes
When reviewing PRO endpoints, regulators expect a clear justification for measuring particular outcomes and the selection of the PRO measure(s) used. The relevance of the chosen outcomes to the therapeutic area and treatment as well as any useful background information from the literature is expect. In addition, regulators also expect a description of how the PRO will fit and work within the clinical development programme in the given patient population. For example, in CNS, relevance and appropriateness of a PRO to the disease stage (early vs. advanced stages) is an important concern. In late stages of disease, it might be challenging to collect information directly from the patient due to cognitive issues.

Further, when dealing with a PRO endpoint's ability to capture treatment effect, besides sensitivity to change in the concept of interest, ability to detect stability (e.g. to be able to identify patient's who are stable) is also important. In patients receiving chemotherapy, for example, it is expected that PROs such as HRQoL, nausea or vitality would worsen or remain constant at best during or following treatment. Regulators want to be sure that the stable or unchanging PRO scores do indeed represent stability in the patient's condition and not a lack of sensitivity to deterioration or improvement.

In order to demonstrate that observed changes in a PRO reflect the patient's clinical status, evidence showing the correlation between the PRO and clinical outcomes was considered crucial to the validity of a PRO measure. This was thought to be lacking for some PRO measures. Closely related to this, the evidence for the 'clinical utility' of the PRO was required, as part of the validity information. Clinical utility was understood as the clinical relevance of the PRO concept being measured or that of a magnitude of a score change in the respective PRO measure, in a specific patient group.

Furthermore, the ability to validly interpret changes in scores of PRO measures was considered crucial; the lack of clear threshold for identifying clinically significant changes taking place was a concern. Such information was expected to be consistent with the trial objectives—superiority, non-inferiority and equivalence. In any case, interpretation of study results became complex where (1) no change was observed, 'does it really mean that the patient's condition did not change or that the PRO measure was not sensitive enough to detect changes', or (2) direction of change differed across the domains of a multidimensional PRO measure. The underlying concern here was whether this was consistent with biological/clinical prognosis of the disease and whether such results were expected and included in the initial design or were surprising or unexpected. In the latter, this leads to many questions on the strength of the PRO measure.

A major challenge in establishing validity of PRO measures in regulatory settings was thought to relate to the difficulty of achieving the ideal situation of a PRO measure validated for every disease, every patient population and every stage of treatment. While guidelines have been developed and presented, they are merely a standard. The approach to be followed in meeting these standards is unclear for the pharmaceutical industry. Moreover, criteria of what evidence is acceptable also remain unclear.

Issues in PRO Interpretation and Application

Various issues related to the clinical trials were also mentioned. This included study design, administration of PRO instruments and the completeness of obtained data. In a bid to incorporate 'something' showing patient benefit, developers tended to add PRO measures as an afterthought rather than in the initial phases of development. This was often reflected in the lack of (1) a thorough conceptualisation of the PRO measured and (2) a statistical analysis plan and criteria for success or failure. Classic examples of this are where 'too many' PRO measures (e.g. up to 14), which are often highly similar and overlapping excessively, were included in clinical trials or situations where PRO measurement strategy is inconsistent with the rest of a trial's objective(s).

Regulators have a strong expectation for double blinding and randomisation in PRO trials. The subjective nature of PROs and the potential confounding of environmental and contextual factors on responses from patients raise major concerns where PROs are obtained using an open-label design. However, this may be a challenge in certain situations, for example, where the drug under study has a high toxicity profile (frequently the case in oncology).

Similar to other endpoints within clinical trials, regulators view incomplete data as a threat to the integrity of study results. The potential confounding between missing data and the outcome of interest (where rates of missing data increased with worse outcome) raised concerns about bias in PRO results with high rates of missing data.

Opportunities for Improving the Generation and Use of PRO Data in Regulatory Processes

- There is a need for the industry to develop consensus on a roadmap and approach for addressing the validity standards of the FDA and the EMA.
- The industry should engage in discussions with the regulators on specific development programmes in terms of the evidence required in establishing validity in relation to specific drug development plans.
- Companies should start thinking about PRO endpoints earlier in the medicines development process, during the design of phase II and phase III studies, rather than shortly before approval or alongside planning for HTA data.
- Regulators have shown an interest and willingness to provide more specific guidance on the suitability/appropriateness of PROs for specific drug development programmes. However, this process needs to be driven by the pharmaceutical industry as regulators are unwilling to do the 'medicines development thinking' on behalf of the industry. They limit their involvement to providing specific feedback and guidance where this is sought. For measures being newly developed, such guidance can be obtained during phase II of a medicines development process. For measures that have already been validated/developed, such consultation can be given later, during phase III.

- A more collaborative approach to instrument development could be adopted, as recently seen in a number of consortiums supported by the drug regulatory agencies.
- A more active role is required of patients and their advocacy groups in leading collaborative efforts to develop PRO measures for specific diseases.

Use of PROs in HTA: An Example of IQWIG and G-BA

Early benefit assessment (EBA) is required within 1 year of launch on the German market, for new drugs eligible for statutory health insurance (SHI) reimbursement. Assessments focus on magnitude of additional patient-relevant benefit in comparison with best available treatment, in terms of mortality and morbidity, i.e. overall survival, health status including severity/duration of disease and HRQoL (IQWIG, 2015). There is still ambiguity regarding relevant outcomes of morbidity and HRQoL and how the right evidence within the EBA procedure looks like. The G-BA, for example, does not consider endpoints such as progression-free survival (PFS) which are widely employed in regulatory procedures as being patient-relevant. For instance, the six morbidity endpoints that appear in the SmPC for obinutuzumab were rejected by the G-BA for lack of patient relevance (Ruof et al. 2014). Further, the G-BA has rejected results on utility measures in favour of single item scores for specific symptoms. Out of 66 EBAs carried out by IQWIG and G-BA as of 2013, 15 dossiers did not include any HRQoL evidence (Lohrberg et al. 2016). HRQoL evidence was pivotal in two positive decisions, relating to crizotinib and ivacaftor (see Box 7.3 for more details on Crizotinib).

Box 7.3 Application of PRO measures in EBA processes, An Example of Crizotinib dossier

Crizotinib is indicated for patients with previously treated anaplastic lymphoma kinase (ALK)-positive advanced lung cancer in whom chemotherapy is indicated. The market authorisation for the drug was based on an open label RCT of oral crizotinib (250 mg) against intravenous chemotherapy in 347 patients, with progression free survival as the primary endpoint (Shaw et al. 2013).

The sponsor's EBA dossier included results from the pivotal trial, where statistically significant benefit was demonstrated on symptoms including pain (chest), cough or dyspnoea assessed using the EORTC QLQ-C30 and the QLQ-LC13 scales, as well as HRQoL assessed using the EORTC QLQ-C30 (disease-specific) and the EQ-5D (generic) (IQWiG, 2013). However, no statistically significant benefit was observed on overall survival.

Based on the evidence submitted, a minor added benefit of crizotinib in terms of dyspnoea, pain and cough symptoms and HRQoL was accepted by IQWIG.

Lohrberg et al. (2016) identified reasons for the low use of HRQoL evidence in EBA assessments, based on their review of EBA dossiers. Key issues identified included (1) differences in conceptualisation of HRQoL between sponsors and IQWIG, (2) lack of significance in study results, (3) poor reporting and presentation of HRQoL results and (4) the overall lack of any HRQoL evidence on a product. Sponsors tended to define HRQoL loosely and widely. The IQWIG rejected concepts such as 'patient satisfaction', 'patient preferences' and 'work productivity' and assessments of QoL by attending physicians. On the other hand, there seemed to be some consensus in considering aspects of treatment burden such as number of daily injections, the need for higher insulin disease and glucose measurement, use of syringes and the need to keep an injection-food delay as aspects of QoL.

More formalised standards and guidance on application of PRO evidence in the G-BA and IQWIGs EBA process would be helpful, given the growing importance of PROs. As a minimum, such guidance ought to include clear definition of conceptual framework, clear delineation of various PRO concepts such as HRQoL and utility, minimal requirements on measurement properties of PRO measures, clinical trial design and criteria for score interpretation and clinical significant change.

Part IV: Current Developments in the Field

The Role of PROs in Facilitating Flexible Regulatory and Access Pathways

A new frontier where PROs are likely to play an instrumental role is in the context of facilitated regulatory and access pathways, which are designed to speed development, market authorisation and patient access to new drugs with a positive benefit-risk balance by providing alternatives to standard product development and regulatory review routes (Liberti et al. 2017). Since 2014, more than half of the NMEs at the FDA were reviewed under some form of FRP (Liberti et al. 2016). Besides shorter review times, evidence used during such review processes is different; surrogate endpoints assume a greater weight, and some of the burden of evidence generation is moved from pre- to post-authorisation phase.

At a recent multi-stakeholder forum (CIRS Workshop; September 2017) bringing together industry, academia and regulators, some of the critical questions at the core of optimisation of FRPs were discussed, including defining criteria for determining which products should be considered for FRPs and FRAPs, identifying issues and opportunities for further alignment/convergence of regulatory and HTA review approaches and processes and addressing different stakeholder perspectives and expectations regarding the outcomes of FRPs.

PROs may be applied in various ways to address these questions. As part of criteria for identifying candidates for FRPs, assessment of unmet medical needs ought to include the patient's perspective – in terms of symptom burden, functional impairment or patient's experiences — and preferences for treatments. Outcomes that are most important to patients could be identified and included in the core outcome set included in post-approval evidence generation, used to address regulatory as well as HTA review data needs. This entails greater methodological alignment between regulatory and HTA workflows, both during study design (scientific advice) and at the review stages.

Regulatory and HTA Scientific Advice

The nature and format of scientific advice offered by the major medicines regulatory agencies such as EMA and FDA are changing. Regulatory agencies now have a more streamlined procedure for providing scientific and protocol assistance to sponsors (European Medicines Agency 2014b), which might be appropriated at any stage of development of a PRO measure. During early development, advice might be sought in relation to a hypothesised conceptual framework, study protocols for planned qualitative research or preliminary data from patients. In later stages, such discussions can be based on detailed results from qualitative work or protocols for quantitative psychometric validation. The level of detail and specificity and the prescriptive nature of such regulatory recommendations on PRO issues have increased. Moreover, patient representatives can now take part in such scientific advice meetings alongside therapeutic area experts.

Initiatives taken by the COAs and OHOP divisions provide a good example of the proactive/prescriptive approach taken by the FDA. The FDA is encouraging assessment of symptomatic adverse events, physical function and disease-related symptoms in all oncology registration trials—using modern measures such as PRO-CTAE and PROMIS PFS. Such an initiative would likely support development of a common framework for measuring PROs in oncology, which would enhance the rigour of PRO data.

Furthermore, starting from 2010, the EMA offers joint scientific advice with HTA agencies. This is meant to ensure that drug developers obtain feedback on the data required for establishing benefit-risk balance and value of drugs from regulators and HTA agencies, respectively, early in the drug development process (European Medicines Agency 2014a). This is intended to streamline both regulatory and HTA procedures, reduce duplication of efforts and potentially minimise the need for additional data collection to address evidential requirements from multiple stakeholders. The relevance of PROs to both the evaluation of efficacy/safety of new medicines and the assessment of their usefulness/benefit to the healthcare system suggests that the joint HTA-EMA parallel scientific advice procedures might be most suitable for PRO measurement and may even encourage greater consideration of PRO claims early in the drug development process.

Regulatory Qualification of Drug Development Tools

Both the EMA and the FDA have created a voluntary pathway for qualifying novel tools used in preclinical and clinical drug development stages as a means to improve the efficiency of drug development and to fast-track the availability of new medicines. Achieving such qualification means that the FDA/EMA has the confidence in the use of such a tool in a specified context, applicable in future drug development scenarios without need for further qualification (European Medicines Agency 2015; US Food and Drug Administration 2014). In case of the EMA, a 'qualification advice' on protocols and study plans can be obtained during early stages of drug development, and the final 'qualification opinion' in later phases. As new PROs intended for use in clinical trial programmes for new medicines are classified as drug development tools, the qualification procedure is equally applicable. At present, 48 clinical outcomes assessment tools (which include PROs) are undergoing the qualification process at the FDA as well as the EMA, with a single PRO measure completing the qualification process: the Exacerbations of Chronic Pulmonary Disease Tool (EXACT) for evaluating the effects of treatment on acute exacerbations of chronic obstructive pulmonary disease (COPD) (European Medicines Agency 2015; US Food and Drug Administration 2014).

The new pathway presents both risks and opportunities. While the qualification process is voluntary, precedence may be set in the future where all PROs applied in drug development must receive such form of approval from the relevant agencies. Although this is unlikely, based on anecdotal evidence, growing tendencies towards a prescriptive approach seen among regulatory agencies is a cause for concern, especially where a PRO label is being sought.

Multi-Stakeholder Approach to PROs

Influential networks and collaborations have emerged involving multiple stakeholders (including the drug development agencies, scientific researchers in health outcomes, clinicians and patient representatives) with the aim of developing publicly available PRO measures to support drug development (Coons et al. 2011). The qualification (previously elaborated) entails that such PRO measures are 'approved' by the regulatory agencies, for measuring given outcomes in specific indications. The Critical Path Institute (C-Path) PRO Consortium is a notable example of such initiatives and draws a wide range of stakeholders as collaborators, including the FDA, the EMA, the US National Institutes of Health and the pharmaceutical industry (http://c-path.org/programs/pro/). Currently, measures are being developed in asthma, cognition, irritable bowel syndrome, depression, lung cancer, functional dyspepsia and rheumatoid arthritis.

The Innovative Medicines Initiative (http://www.imi.europa.eu/content/mission), supported by the European Federation of Pharmaceutical Industries and Associations (EFPIA) and the European Commission, is an example of such collaborations within Europe. Specifically, the PRO-Active consortium is developing PRO measures for assessing physical activity and symptoms in COPD.

Recently, the FDA has compiled a compendium summarising how COA information has been used in registration trials, labelling claims as well as qualified COAs. The current version of the compendium is in a pilot phase and includes information 144 COA reviews, based on drug labelling approved from 2003 to 2014. Information reported includes disease/condition, indication and/or description of claim, COA outcome of interest, COA type, COA context of use and COA qualification information. This tool is likely to be highly useful to researchers and sponsors in designing COA aspects of registration trials, particularly reducing the overhead resources required in designing studies/selection of appropriate COA measures.

A collaborative approach to instrument development has both a practical and a scientific significance. The involvement of multiple stakeholders and consideration of multiple perspectives in the design of the measure development process are likely to improve the rigour and quality of the resultant measure. The involvement of regulatory agencies also entails a greater chance of fulfilling regulatory requirements on PRO measures. On the other hand, this is also likely to encourage and foster consensus on the definition of outcomes within a particular disease condition with drug development programmes. From a practical point of view, consortia would avail more resource (human and financial) facilitating implementation of the most appropriate study designs.

Technology and Communication Revolution

Numerous smart wearable sensors (SWS) such as accelerometers and gyroscopes are now available for medical as well as general health use. SWS are transforming the monitoring of physiological outcomes, making it possible to gather objective data on outcomes which would have previously solely relied on PROs. For example, in neurological monitoring, SWS with capabilities to analyse gait, length and step count have shown potential in limb paralysis and assessment of cerebral palsy PD and AD.

Online patient social networks have now become more dynamic—employing various forms of social media channels – and have given rise to new forms of data. For example, within outcomes research/PRO research, social media is being used for (1) recruitment of patients especially in rare diseases, (2) investigation of health status and behaviours related to treatment and (3) public evaluation of symptoms and effectiveness of treatments (http://curetogether.com/blog/about/) and as (4) a rich source of insight into the views of patients on their disease experiences and on their treatments (Gustafson and Woodworth 2014).

References

Beckman HB, Frankel RM (1984) The effect of physician behavior on the collection of data. Ann Intern Med 101(5):692–696

Boers M, Kirwan JR, Wells G, Beaton D, Gossec L, d'Agostino M-A, Conaghan PG, Bingham CO, Brooks P, Landewé R (2014) Developing Core outcome measurement sets for clinical trials: OMERACT filter 2.0. J Clin Epidemiol 67(7):745–753

Brundage MD, Smith KC, Little EA, Bantug ET, Snyder CF (2015) Communicating patient-reported outcome scores using graphic formats: results from a mixed-methods evaluation. Qual Life Res 24(10):2457–2472

Calkins DR, Rubenstein LV, Cleary PD, Davies AR, Jette AM, Fink A, Kosecoff J, Young RT, Brook RH, Delbanco TL (1991) Failure of physicians to recognize functional disability in ambulatory patients. Ann Intern Med 114(6):451–454

Calvert M, Blazeby J, Altman DG, Revicki DA, Moher D, Brundage MD, CONSORT PRO Group (2013a) Reporting of patient-reported outcomes in randomized trials: the CONSORT PRO extension. JAMA 309(8):814–822

Calvert M, Brundage M, Jacobsen PB, Schünemann HJ, Efficace F (2013b) The CONSORT patient-reported outcome (PRO) extension: implications for clinical trials and practice. Health Qual Life Outcomes 11(1):184

Clark MJ, Harris N, Griebsch I, Kaschinski D, Copley-Merriman C (2014) Patient-reported outcome labeling claims and measurement approach for metastatic castration-resistant prostate Cancer treatments in the United States and European Union. Health Qual Life Outcomes 12(1):104

Cohen SR, Boston P, Mount BM, Porterfield P (2001) Changes in quality of life following admission to palliative care units. Palliat Med 15(5):363–371

Cohen SR, Mount BM (2000) Living with Cancer:'good' days and 'bad' days—what produces them? Cancer 89(8):1854–1865

Coons SJ, Kothari S, Monz BU, Burke LB (2011) The patient-reported outcome (PRO) consortium: filling measurement gaps for PRO end points to support labeling claims. Clin Pharmacol Ther 90(5):743–748

DeMuro C, Clark M, Mordin M, Fehnel S, Copley-Merriman C, Gnanasakthy A (2013) Reasons for rejection of patient-reported outcome label claims: a compilation based on a review of patient-reported outcome use among new molecular entities and biologic license applications, 2006–2010. Value Health 15(3):443–448

Detmar SB, Aaronson NK (1998) Quality of life assessment in daily clinical oncology practice: a feasibility study. Eur J Cancer 34(8):1181–1186

Detmar SB, Muller MJ, Schornagel JH, Wever LDV, Aaronson NK (2002) Health-related quality-of-life assessments and patient-physician communication: a randomized controlled trial. JAMA 288(23):3027–3034

Deyo RA, Carter WB (1992) Strategies for improving and expanding the application of health status measures in clinical settings: a researcher-developer viewpoint. Med Care 30:MS176–MS186

Efficace F, Feuerstein M, Fayers P, Cafaro V, Eastham J, Pusic A, Blazeby J, EORTC Quality of Life Group (2014) Patient-reported outcomes in randomised controlled trials of prostate Cancer: methodological quality and impact on clinical decision making. Eur Urol 66(3):416–427

European Medicines Agency (2014a) Best practice guidance for pilot EMA HTA parallel scientific advice procedures. European Medicines Agency, London

European Medicines Agency (2014b) European medicines agency guidance for applicants seeking scientific advice and protocol assistance. European Medicines Agency, London

European Medicines Agency (2015) EMA/CHMP/SAWP/178465/2015. Draft qualification opinion of qualification of exacerbations of chronic pulmonary disease tool (EXACT), and EXACT- respiratory symptoms measure (E-RS) for evaluating treatment outcomes in clinical trials in COPD. European Medicines Agency, London

Fayers PM, Machin D (2007) Scores and measurements: validity, reliability, sensitivity. In: Quality of life. John Wiley & Sons, Ltd, Hoboken, pp 77–108. https://doi.org/10.1002/9780470024522.ch4

Gnanasakthy A, DeMuro C, Clark M, Mordin M, Thomas S (2013a) Role of patient-reported outcome measures in the assessment of central nervous system agents. Ther Innov Regul Sci 47(5):613–618

Gnanasakthy A, Lewis S, Clark M, Mordin M, DeMuro C (2013b) Potential of patient-reported outcomes as Nonprimary endpoints in clinical trials. Health Qual Life Outcomes 11(1):83. https://doi.org/10.1186/1477-7525-11-83

Gnanasakthy A, DeMuro C, Boulton C (2013c) Integration of patient-reported outcomes in multiregional confirmatory clinical trials. Contemp Clin Trials 35(1):62–69

Greenhalgh J, Long AF, Flynn R (2005) The use of patient reported outcome measures in routine clinical practice: lack of impact or lack of theory? Soc Sci Med 60(4):833–843

Gustafson DL, Woodworth CF (2014) Methodological and ethical issues in research using social media: a Metamethod of human papillomavirus vaccine studies. BMC Med Res Methodol 14(1):127

Hao Y (2010) Patient-reported outcomes in support of oncology product labeling claims: regulatory context and challenges. Expert Rev Pharmacoecon Outcomes Res 10(4):407–420

Higginson IJ, Carr AJ (2001) Measuring quality of life: using quality of life measures in the clinical setting. BMJ 322(7297):1297

Institute For Quality and Efficiency in Healthcare (2013) Crizotinib: Benefit Assessment According to § 35a SGB V Social Code Book. Dossier Assessment A12-15. Extract IQWiG-Report No. 151. https://www.iqwig.de/download/A12-15_Crizotinib_%20Extract-of-dossier-assessment.pdf. Accessed 23 Jan 2018

Institute For Quality And Efficiency In Health Care. (2015). General methods. Version 4.2 (English Version). https://www.iqwig.de/download/IQWiG_General_Methods_Version_%204-2.pdf. Accessed 23 Jan 2018

Koller M, Klinkhammer-Schalke M, Lorenz W (2005) Outcome and quality of life in medicine: a conceptual framework to put quality of life research into practice, vol 23. Elsevier, Amsterdam, pp 186–192

Liberti L, Breckenridge A, Hoekman J, Leufkens H, Lumpkin M, McAuslane N, Stolk P, Zhi K, Rägo L (2016) Accelerating access to new medicines: current status of facilitated regulatory pathways used by emerging regulatory authorities. J Public Health Policy 37(3):315–333

Liberti L, Bujar M, Breckenridge A, Hoekman J, McAuslane N, Stolk P, Leufkens H (2017) FDA facilitated regulatory pathways: visualizing their characteristics, development, and authorization timelines. Front Pharmacol 8:161

Lohrberg D, Augustin M, Blome C (2016) The definition and role of quality of life in Germany's early assessment of drug benefit: a qualitative approach. Qual Life Res 25(2):447–455

Pratheepawanit N, Salek MS, Finlay IG (1999) The applicability of quality-of-life assessment in palliative care: comparing two quality-of-life measures. Palliat Med 13(4):325–334

Cohen SR, Mount BM, Bruera E, Provost M, Rowe J, Tong K (1997) Validity of the McGill quality of life questionnaire in the palliative care setting: a multi-centre Canadian study demonstrating the importance of the existential domain. Palliat Med 11(1):3–20

Ruof J, Knoerzer D, Dünne A-A, Dintsios C-M, Staab T, Schwartz FW (2014) Analysis of endpoints used in marketing authorisations versus value assessments of oncology medicines in Germany. Health Policy 118(2):242–254

Schor EL, Lerner DJ, Malspeis S (1995) Physicians' assessment of functional health status and well-being: the Patient's perspective. Arch Intern Med 155(3):309–314

Shaw AT, Kim DW, Nakagawa K, Seto T, Crinó L, Ahn MJ, De Pas T, Besse B, Solomon BJ, Blackhall F, Wu YL (2013) Crizotinib versus chemotherapy in advanced ALK-positive lung cancer. N Engl J Med 368(25):2385–2394

Siminoff LA, Fetting JH, Abeloff MD (1989) Doctor-patient communication about breast Cancer adjuvant therapy. J Clin Oncol 7(9):1192–1200

Snyder CF, Herman JM, White SM, Luber BS, Blackford AL, Carducci MA, Wu AW (2014) When using patient-reported outcomes in clinical practice, the measure matters: a randomized controlled trial. J Oncol Pract 10(5):e299–e306

Snyder CF, Smith KC, Bantug ET, Tolbert EE, Blackford AL, Brundage MD (2017) What do these scores mean? Presenting patient-reported outcomes data to patients and clinicians to improve interpretability. Cancer 123(10):1848–1859

US Food and Drug Administration (2014) Draft guidance for industry on qualification of exacerbations of chronic pulmonary disease tool for measurement of symptoms of acute bacterial exacerbation of chronic bronchitis in patients with chronic obstructive pulmonary disease. Fed Regist 79:1873

Valderas JM, Rue M, Guyatt G, Alonso J (2005) The impact of the VF-14 index, a perceived visual function measure, in the routine Management of Cataract Patients. Qual Life Res 14(7):1743–1753

Velikova G, Booth L, Smith AB, Brown PM, Lynch P, Brown JM, Selby PJ (2004) Measuring quality of life in routine oncology practice improves communication and patient well-being: a randomized controlled trial. J Clin Oncol 22(4):714–724

Wagner AK, Vickrey BG (1995) The routine use of health-related quality of life measures in the Care of Patients with epilepsy: rationale and research agenda. Qual Life Res 4(2):169–177

Wild D, Eremenco S, Mear I, Martin M, Houchin C, Gawlicki M, Hareendran A, Wiklund I, Chong LY, Von Maltzahn R (2009) Multinational trials—recommendations on the translations required, approaches to using the same language in different countries, and the approaches to support pooling the data: the ISPOR patient-reported outcomes translation and linguistic validation good research practices task force report. Value Health 12(4):430–440

Wild D, Grove A, Martin M, Eremenco S, McElroy S, Verjee-Lorenz A, Erikson P (2005) Principles of good practice for the translation and cultural adaptation process for patient-reported outcomes (PRO) measures: report of the ISPOR task force for translation and cultural adaptation. Value Health 8(2):94–104

MIX
Papier aus verantwortungsvollen Quellen
Paper from responsible sources
FSC® C105338
FSC
www.fsc.org

If you have any concerns about our products,
you can contact us on
ProductSafety@springernature.com

In case Publisher is established outside the EU,
the EU authorized representative is:
Springer Nature Customer Service Center GmbH
Europaplatz 3, 69115 Heidelberg, Germany

Printed by Libri Plureos GmbH
in Hamburg, Germany